Orgasms

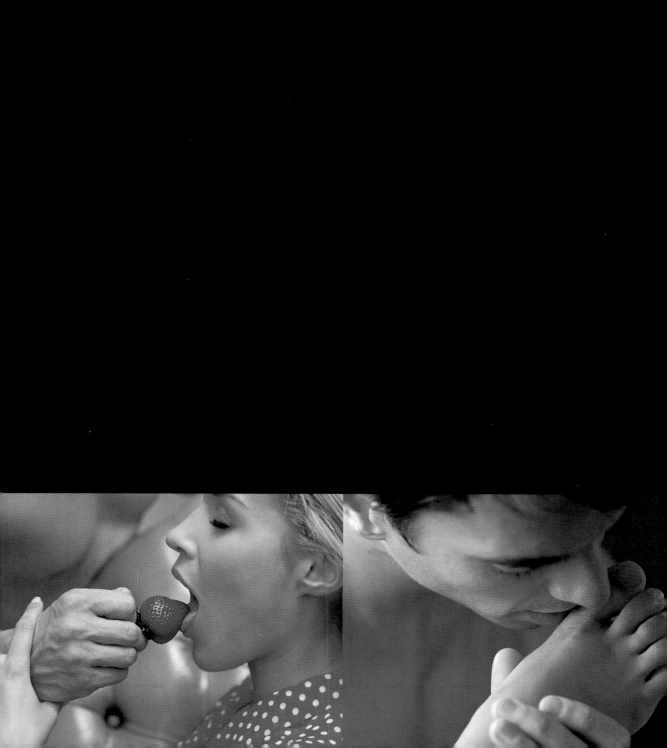

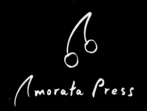

Amorata Press

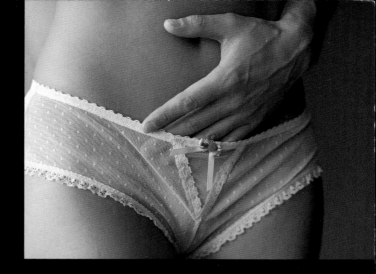

Orgasms

A Sensual Guide to Female Ecstasy

Nicci Talbot

Published in the U.S. by
AMORATA PRESS,
an imprint of Ulysses Press
P.O. Box 3440
Berkeley, CA 94703
www.amoratapress.com

First published in Great Britain in 2007 by
Hamlyn, a division of Octopus Publishing Group Ltd.

ISBN10: 1-56975-580-9
ISBN13: 978-1-56975-580-8
Library of Congress Catalog Number: 2006907917

Printed and bound in China
10 9 8 7 6 5 4 3 2 1

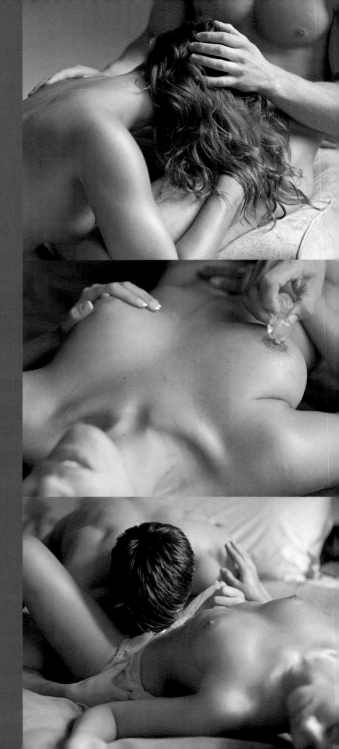

Contents

Introduction

Ever wondered what happens to your body during an orgasm? Or why it is easier to have one at certain times of the month? Did you know that men and women are capable of experiencing at least six different kinds of orgasm? And that you can have one lasting up to three hours? Welcome to *Orgasms*, the book that is all about you and your orgasms!

Orgasms are fantastic

Orgasms are a vital part of our sexual growth and a basic human need. Psychoanalyst Wilhelm Reich first linked orgasm to mental health in 1927, in his book *The Function of the Orgasm*, and defined neurosis as blocks to having a full orgasm. Never mind an apple a day: an orgasm a day circulates energy around the body, increases your heart rate and relieves you of stress and tension.

And yet orgasms are such a great source of angst. In movies everyone is having mind-blowing multiples. Who could blame us for wondering if we're doing something wrong? For something that's supposed to be fun they certainly stir up a lot of anxiety and worry.

There's hope yet!

The good news is that you can improve your orgasms – and this book shows you how. It's simply a matter of knowing how your body works. The more you explore your sexuality and learn about orgasms, the better your orgasms will be. This is definitely one thing that improves with age. The first part of the book, "Understanding Orgasm," is an exploration of what an orgasm actually is, why it is good for you and what happens to your body and brain when you climax. "Exploring Your Body" goes on to uncover those important parts – the clitoris and the G-spot – that make orgasm such a sensual experience and has some great tips for fabulous solo sex. It also shows you how to indulge in a little sexual foreplay with your partner through fantasy, aphrodisiacs, dressing up and dressing down, as well as oral stimulation and erotic massage.

"Experiencing Orgasm" is all about achieving that long-awaited climax – with and without intercourse. Here you discover the many ways you can reach orgasm and the best positions for prolonging the pleasure. There's also an insight into the spiritual sex theories of Tantra, Tao and the *Kama Sutra*.

Sexual problems are not overlooked – let's face it, no one has the perfect relationship – so there's lots of information about the physical and psychological factors that can kill your libido and what you can do about them.

Keep this book by your bedside rather than on the bookshelf and it shouldn't be long before it is well-thumbed and smeared with massage oil.

Have fun!

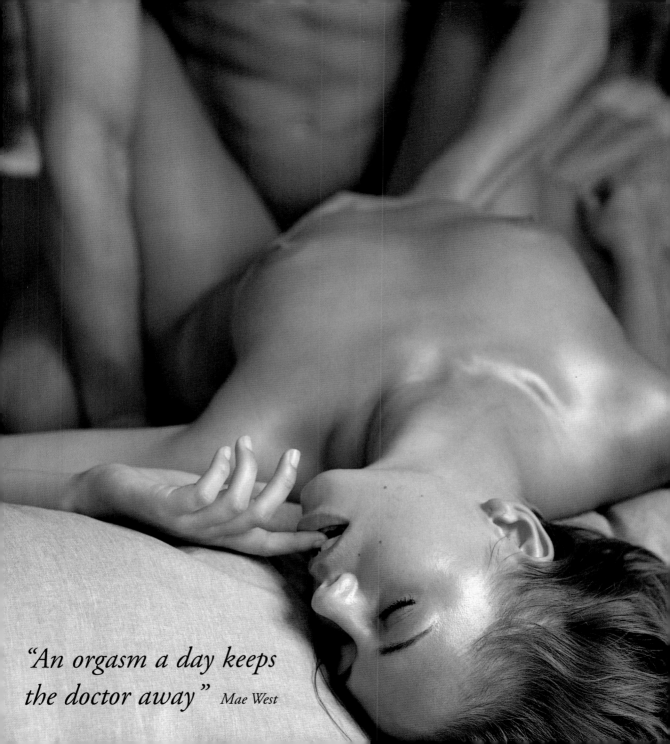

*"An orgasm a day keeps
the doctor away"* Mae West

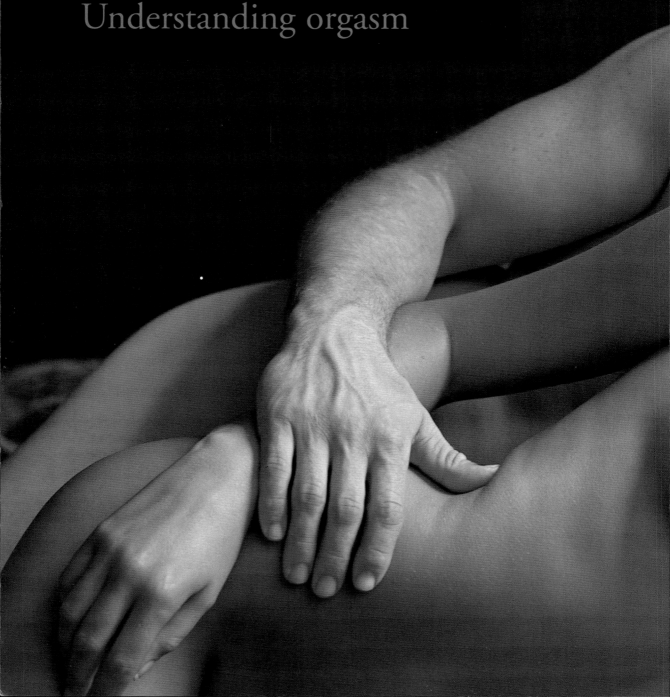

Understanding orgasm

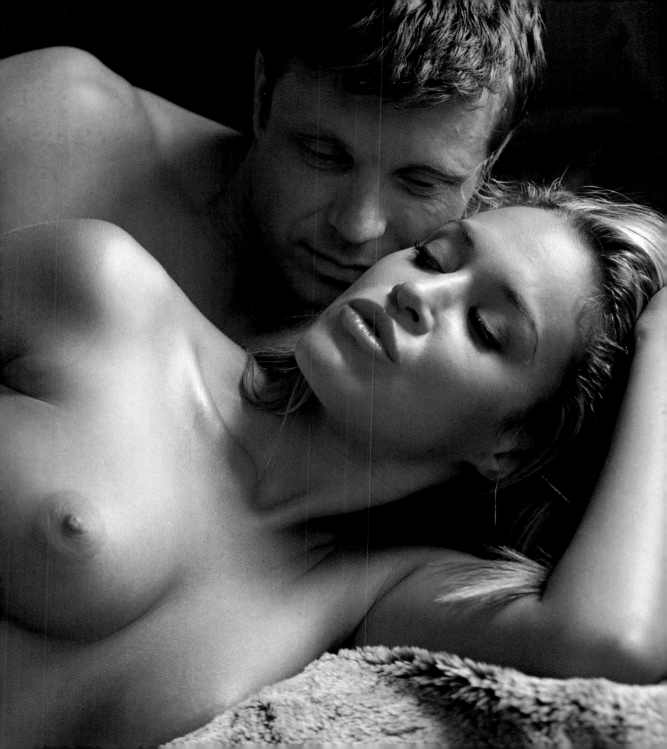

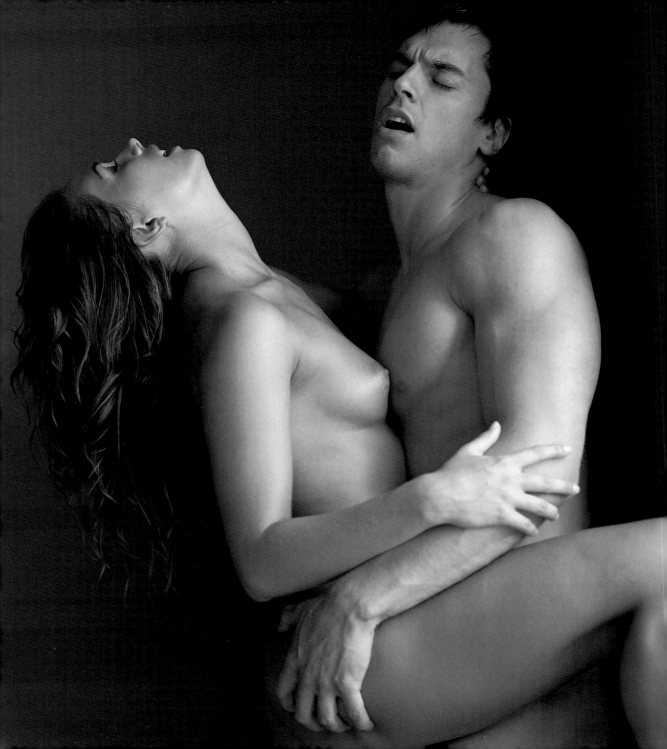

What is an orgasm?

The word orgasm comes from the Greek word *orgasmós*, which means to swell; be lustful. What you experience when you have an orgasm is a physical, psychological and emotional response to sexual stimulation. Orgasms happen when your body can't take any more and simply has to let go.

So what happens?

William Howell Masters and Virginia Eshelman Johnson, who pioneered sex research in the United States during the 1950s and 1960s, described orgasm as a muscular and hydraulic process. Orgasm is the third stage of four in Masters and Johnson's "human sexual response cycle" (see pages 14–17). The experience of this cycle is similar in both sexes, peaking with a series of rhythmic contractions. Men usually ejaculate when they orgasm and experience it primarily in their genitals. Women can experience orgasm in different parts of the body – they can even achieve a whole-body orgasm (see page 94). According to sexpert Tracey Cox, there is no standard "type": An orgasm may be a tiny flutter or an earth-shattering eruption; it may be super-quick or drawn out.

Orgasm is an experience of mind, body and spirit

You and your orgasms

Masters and Johnson's mechanical analysis of orgasm leaves little room for romance, let alone any emotion. It may be more helpful to see orgasm as something that is influenced by your feelings and spiritual state, as well as your body. If you open your mind to new techniques and practices, you may experience sensations you never imagined.

Orgasms are something personal to treasure, look forward to and have fun with. The secret is to never put too much pressure on yourself to have one: They are not the be-all and end-all of sex. They are simply part of an active sex life. Unlike in the movies, real sex is not always orgasmic – and that's fine. There will be certain times of the month when your body is less responsive to touch and other times when the slightest stimulation drives you wild. This is because your desire and ability to orgasm are affected by ovulation. Put simply, a woman feels most like having sex just before ovulating, because this is when she is at her most fertile.

Changing attitudes towards orgasm

There is a prevailing attitude in the West that an orgasm is the pinnacle of sex. It is the supreme goal and if we don't achieve it, we feel that we are somehow failing. We are bombarded by imagery of gorgeous couples engrossed in great sex and it's hard to live up to that. No wonder we feel a little inadequate at times!

Different approaches

In Eastern cultures, however, attitudes towards orgasm can be entirely different. In the Tantra, Tao and *Kama Sutra* traditions (see pages 116–133), an orgasm isn't a sexual target, but a sacred, spiritual and integral part of a much wider sexual experience. Paradoxically, by taking the focus off orgasm and reducing the pressure to perform, the sexual techniques of these traditions can make reaching orgasm easier for some people.

Sex and the past

Historically, female sexuality has had bad press. In the Middle Ages, it was seen as evil and something to be feared. Women weren't supposed to have sex for their own pleasure and female arousal was often viewed as a mental illness, with symptoms that included being wet, thinking about sex and behaving erratically. The vibrator was actually invented as a means to cure female patients of this "hysteria" – an intriguing challenge for bored doctors who had to "relieve" their female patients!

By the 18th century, there was some understanding of the clitoris's role during sex, but the advance of knowledge was hampered somewhat by Sigmund Freud. In the 1920s, he dismissed clitoral orgasms as "immature," claiming that real women had vaginal orgasms. The clitoral orgasm resurfaced again during the 1950s and 1960s, thanks to Alfred Kinsey and his team of researchers. Following this work, Masters and Johnson did much to establish the theories about desire, sex and orgasms that we rely on today.

We have continued to explore female sexuality, establishing, for example, that the clitoris is actually much bigger than was at first thought (see page 30). Another important discovery was the G-spot, which spawned a whole new sexual debate (see page 32). One thing's for sure: Discussion about female sexuality and orgasm has never been dull!

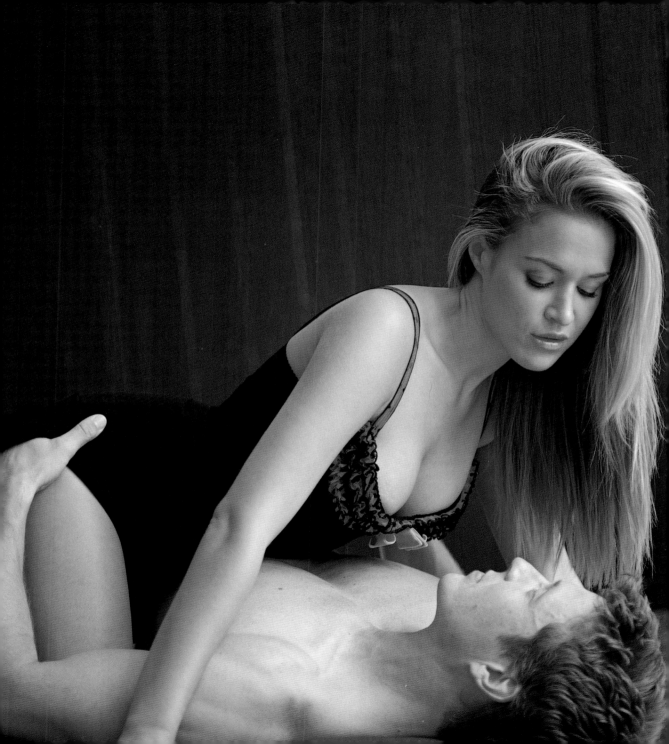

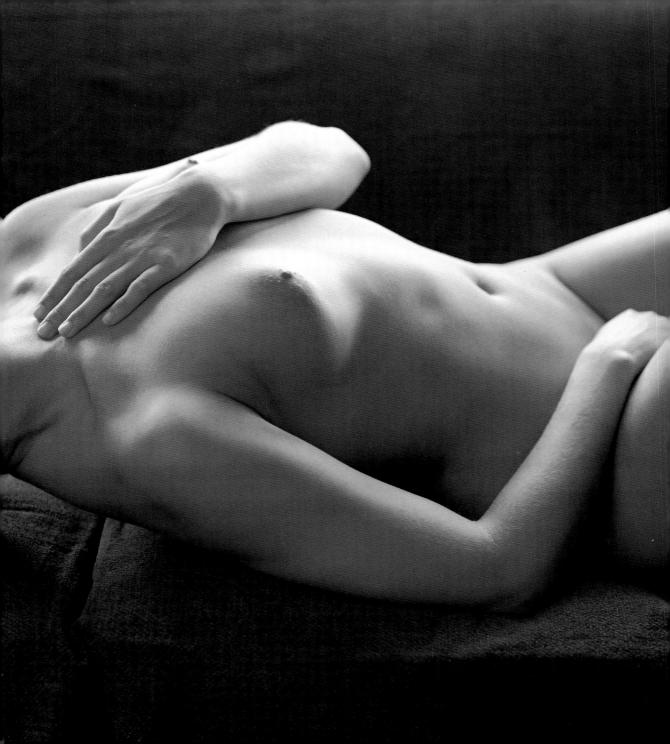

The human sexual response cycle

It's important to know exactly what happens to your body during arousal and orgasm. Lack of libido is the number one complaint among many women, according to sex therapists. Understanding your sexual response and what turns you on can help you to improve your sex drive. So how does it work?

Four stages of response

Sexologists Masters and Johnson defined four stages of physiological response during sexual stimulation, outlining roughly what happens to your body from the moment you first think about sex to the point of orgasm and immediately afterwards. Although this scheme is widely accepted, it is important to remember that your sexual response also depends on some other factors – your mood, how turned on you are, even how you feel about your partner.

1: Excitement

Stimulation can be physical or mental – touching, kissing, having a kinky thought or reading something that turns you on. In response to these thoughts and sensations, the brain triggers an increase of blood in the body and you begin to gear up for sex. Your heart and breathing rates increase and your blood pressure rises. Your nipples have a

mini-erection, as do your man's. You get that rosy glow and he might get it too, a flush that moves up from the tummy to the chest. You sweat on your forehead, upper lip, chest, thighs and ankles. Best of all, your muscle tone increases in some areas.

Once a man's brain registers that it's turned on, it sends a message to his penis, which causes blood to flow to the tissues, making the penis stiff. His erection might come and go. His testes are drawn snug and his scrotum gets thicker.

It can take women up to 45 minutes to get really turned on. That's why lots of foreplay is essential. When you are turned on, your nipples become fully erect and your breasts swollen. Your labia majora (vaginal outer lips) become flatter, thinner and move up and out, increasing in size. Your labia minora (vaginal inner lips) also get larger. Your clitoris has its own mini-erection and the vagina starts to lubricate in preparation for sex. It also changes shape slightly, stretching to accommodate the penis.

2: Plateau

This is the period just before orgasm. Your heart rate and blood circulation increase further, you sweat more and blood rushes to your genitals. At this point you will be ultra-sensitive to touch.

Men tend to get excited pretty quickly and then have a longer plateau before orgasm. The muscles at the base of the penis start contracting, the glans swells and the testicles sit even more snugly next to the body. At this point their heart rate doubles to around 180 beats per minute.

In women, the plateau stage is shorter. Your labia minora swell further and your clitoris moves away from the body. Your pubococcygeus (PC) muscle gets tighter and your breathing rate almost matches his.

3: Orgasm

When it all gets too much, your body explodes into orgasm, releasing the tension. Both sexes have contractions in the anus and pelvic area at around 0.8 seconds apart. You experience lots of lovely body spasms and feel damned good! His orgasm lasts around 5 seconds, and yours about 15.

In men, the processes of orgasm and ejaculation are separate, which means that he can come without having an orgasm. He feels contractions in his penis and knows that he's about to come – physically, he cannot stop himself. His pelvic muscles contract, making fluid move through the urethra. Semen spurts out of the tip of the penis, the amount depending on how long it's been since he last had an orgasm, how old he is and how healthy.

In a woman, the vagina expands at the point of orgasm, the clitoris moves back under its hood and the uterus contracts slightly, causing the cervix to dip into the semen, now in the vaginal area. Unlike men, women can hold off on climaxing until they are ready and are also able to come more than once in succession (see page 82).

4: Resolution

After orgasm, your muscles relax and blood pressure and breathing return to normal. You will both be blissfully exhausted thanks to the release of the hormone prolactin, secreted in the pituitary gland.

For a man, resolution is usually quick. He goes into a refractory period and the penis becomes limp and shrinks to half its erect size. The testicles drop and, quite often, he is soon asleep!

In a woman, resolution means that the cervix opens and blood flow to the nipples and genitals lessens. These areas can remain excited after orgasm, leading to the possibility of multiples.

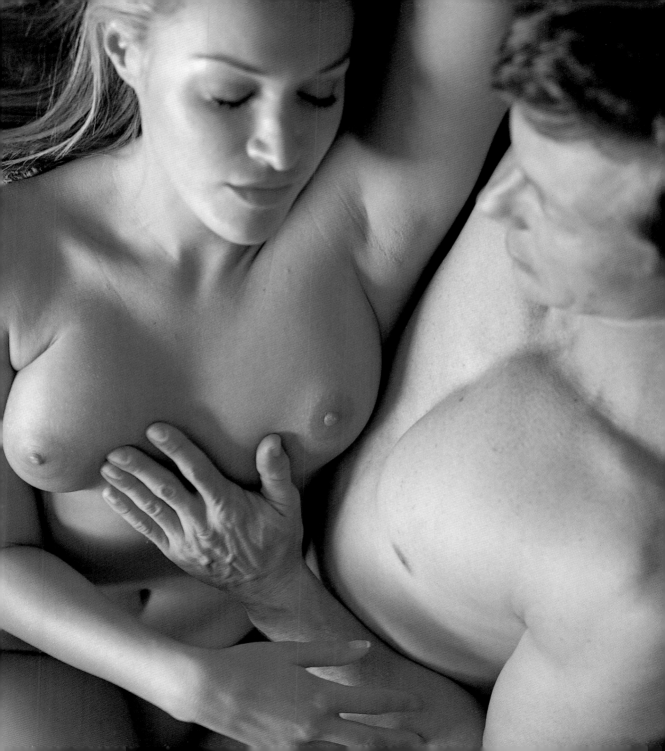

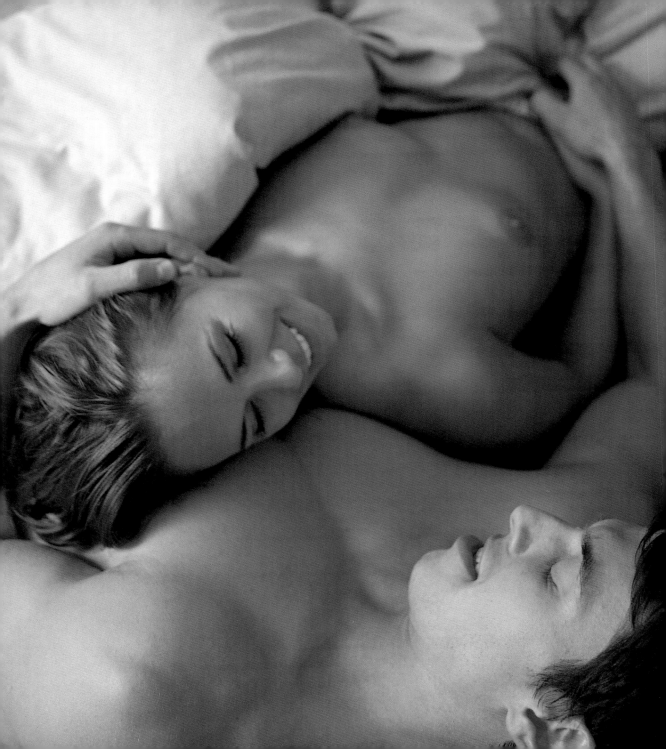

Orgasms are good for you

It's well known that orgasms relieve tension, making you happier and more relaxed. They are a wonderful natural cure for stress and insomnia. But do you know what else your orgasms can do for you?

Health benefits

There's lots of scientific evidence about the amazing effects that orgasms and regular sex can have on your health and well-being. Studies have found that sexually active people live longer and take less time off work; that having sex three times a week can make us look 10 years younger; and that the more a man orgasms, the less likely he is to develop prostate cancer. Yet another study has shown that orgasms can even cure migraines: of 52 sufferers in the study, 16 reported relief from pain when they had an orgasm and 8 said that their headache disappeared altogether. Best of all, it seems that orgasms enhance the libido – the more of them you have, the more you want!

And there's more…

- **Orgasm boosts levels of serotonin**, which is vital for all-around good health, happiness and well-being.
- **Orgasm improves circulation** and makes tissues and organs healthier.
- **During orgasm your body** produces phenetylamine, a natural chemical that controls appetite. You may find yourself losing your cravings for junk food.
- **You produce testosterone** when you orgasm, which helps to protect your heart.
- **Your muscles tighten** during orgasm, so you're toning without having to hit the gym.
- **Even the male orgasm** is good for women; semen is said to contain hormones that lessen depression.
- **Orgasm may increase** the chances of conception. During orgasm, vaginal contractions pull in the sperm, guiding it towards the egg.

Can't come, won't come

With so much pressure to have great orgasms, it is hardly surprising that women (and men) sometimes fake it. Not coming can be a real let-down, making you feel as though you're not having sex properly or you don't know how to satisfy your partner. If you are faking it because you really can't come, don't shrug it off. Get the problem looked into because there is probably a physical or psychological cause that can be overcome (see page 23 for some likely underlying causes).

Sexual dysfunction

Anorgasmia is an inability to orgasm. It affects women at different levels: primary, when a woman has never reached orgasm; secondary, when she once did but no longer does; and situational, when she is able to reach orgasm in certain situations (such as masturbation) but not during others (such as intercourse). The problem is linked to an inability to "let go" during sex, and can be both a medical and psychological problem.

Vaginismus is an inability to handle penetration. The pubococcygeus (PC) muscle surrounding the entrance to the vagina contracts involuntarily, making penetration painful, even impossible. It can occur the first time a woman has sex or it may develop furthur along in a relationship. As with anorgasmia, the reasons for the condition can be physical or psychological.

Erectile dysfunction is an inability to get and maintain an erection during sex. This is quite common, and seems to worsen with age. Although it happens to most men at some stage, and is easily overcome, if it becomes a psychological problem (because he worries about it) it can lead to loss of libido and erection altogether. This is a difficulty that can affect both partners in the relationship, leaving the man feeling ashamed, and the woman rejected and undesired.

Premature ejaculation means coming too soon, usually within moments of penetration. This is a very common sexual complaint and is only an issue if it's causing either partner distress, perhaps if the man begins to feel that he is not a "real man," or the woman becomes frustrated by repeated occurrences.

Sexual anhedonia means that the man experiences erection and ejaculation but cannot orgasm. This is usually associated with a lack of interest in sex.

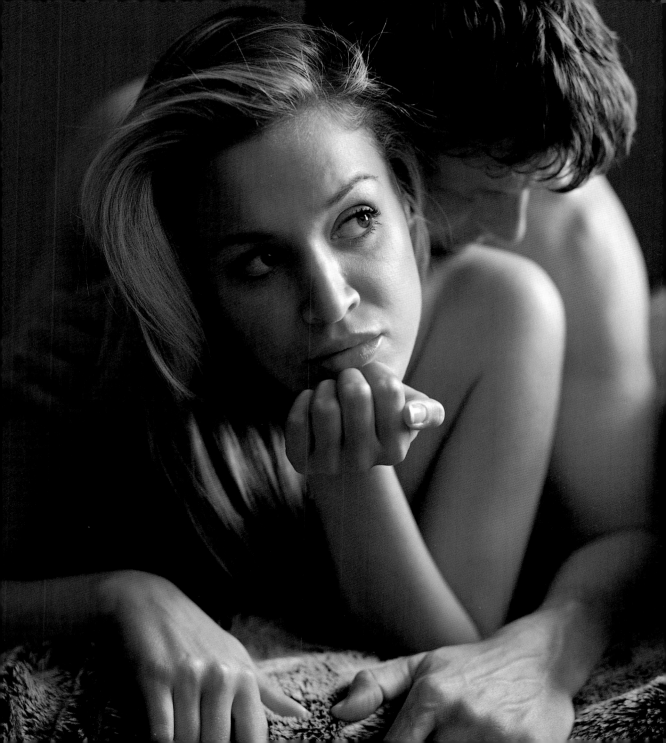

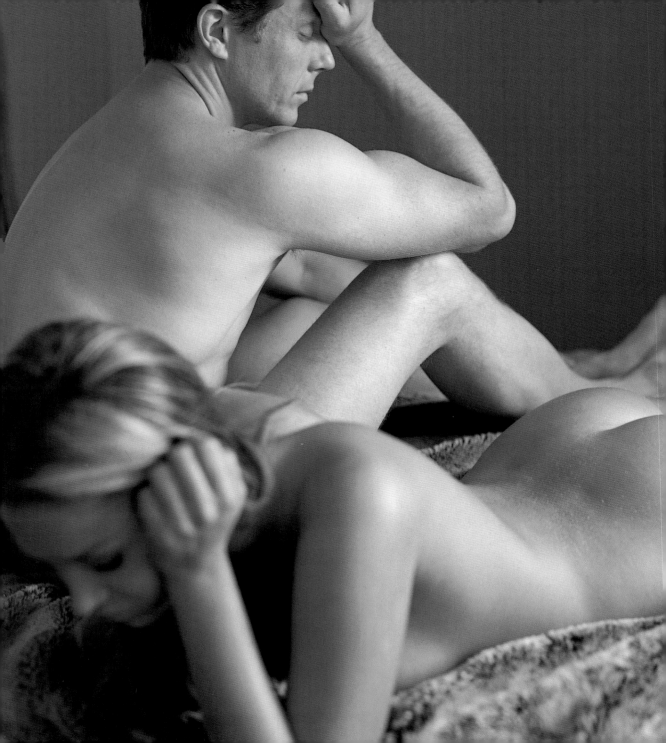

Physical causes

- **Mismatched libidos.** You might want more sex than your partner does, or vice versa; he might want it in the morning while you might be more of a night owl.
- **Lack of foreplay.** You may simply not be ready for sex. Men tend to get turned on more quickly than women. Without sufficient foreplay, you might end up feeling dry, making sex painful, which can leave you unable to orgasm. You may also feel resentment and frustration, imagining that sex is for your partner's gratification alone.
- **Poor sexual technique.** Inadequate thrusting or being too vigorous, rushing sex, or always having sex in the same position, time and location can all be a real turn-off.
- **Excessive use of alcohol or drugs.** Your inhibitions may be lowered initially, but your sexual response will be slowed. Alcohol also dehydrates the body, which could make sex uncomfortable.
- **Certain medical conditions.** Diabetes in men can harden and narrow the arteries, reducing blood flow to the penis and genitals. In women, poor blood circulation, lack of development in the PC muscles or spinal injury can be the cause of sexual dysfunction.

Barriers to
orgasm

Some common causes of sexual dysfunction are described here (for solutions, see page 138). There may be an underlying physical or medical problem, or it may simply be that the brain is getting in the way of sexual pleasure: Overanalyzing can make orgasm less likely.

Psychological causes

There are many reasons why you might find it difficult to relax and enjoy the moment for what it is. You might feel self-conscious about your appearance or be afraid of losing control – remember that orgasm is about trust and self-expression and you can't control how it happens.

While having sex with a non-expressive partner can diminish your sexual confidence, a new sexual partner can also bring a range of insecurities and fears. You may wonder what he will think of your body or sexual technique, and how you compare to previous lovers.

Another barrier to orgasm is being too focused on the event itself. Placing too great an emphasis on having an orgasm – treating it as a goal to attain through sex – can make it unachievable.

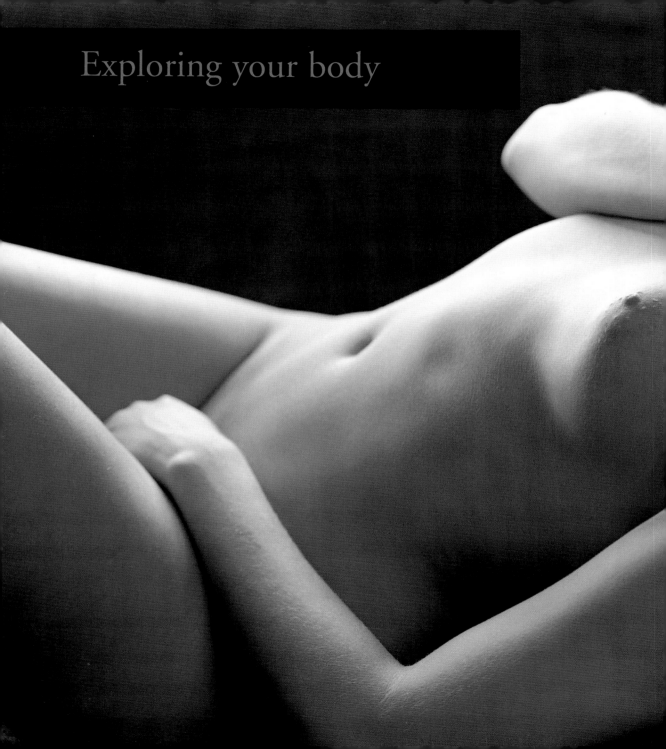

Exploring your body

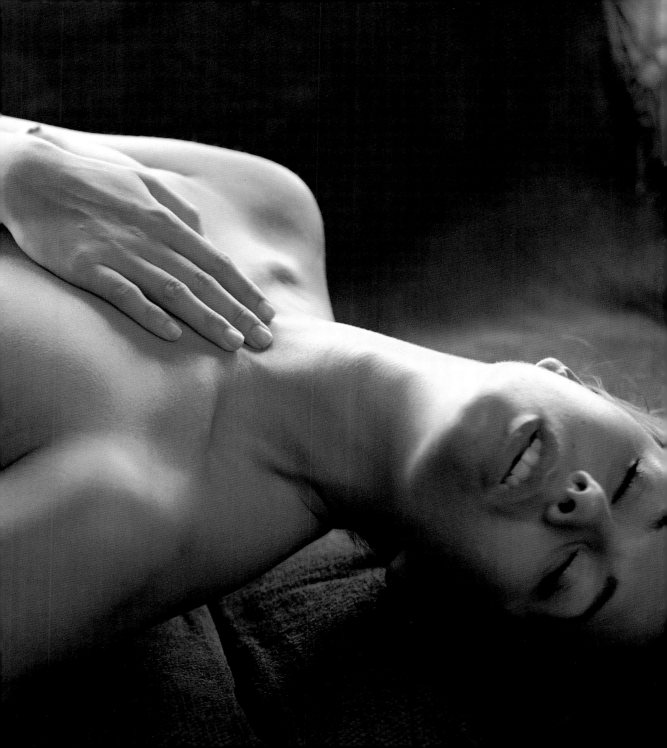

Solo sex

How can you expect your partner to know what makes you orgasm if you don't know yourself? It is only by exploring your body intimately that you can find out what works for you, and most of us learn this through solo sex. Why? Because we have fewer inhibitions when we're doing it alone, we make more time for ourselves and we are more likely to relax properly.

It'll do you good!

The great thing about solo sex is that it is harmless; it's the safest form of sex possible. And yet, in some cultures and religions it still has a stigma, which means that many people don't do it because they feel inhibited or guilty, or think it's a sin. Back in Victorian times, masturbation was considered a perversion and a cause of insanity. Things might have improved today but it still isn't a topic we discuss openly. That's a shame, because solo sex keeps you ticking down below: The more sex you have, and the more you orgasm, the more orgasms you want and the more your body learns to expect. And orgasm is good for you – physically, mentally and spiritually.

"Don't knock it – it's sex with someone I love" Woody Allen

So what are you waiting for?

Love yourself regularly and you will look better, feel more alive and have better concentration levels. That rosy afterglow also makes you irresistible to the opposite sex. "Is there something different about you? You look really healthy!" Men definitely pick up on these things. It's almost as if your body is sending out a subconscious message telling them that you want to play!

Once you know exactly what floats your boat, you can let your partner know. He will enjoy sex all the more if he knows for sure that he is giving you pleasure. Plus, really turning each other on will strengthen your relationship in and out of bed. If you like the idea, try masturbating in front of each other. It can be a huge turn-on, and you'll both find out exactly what strokes to make and how firm to be when you do it to each other.

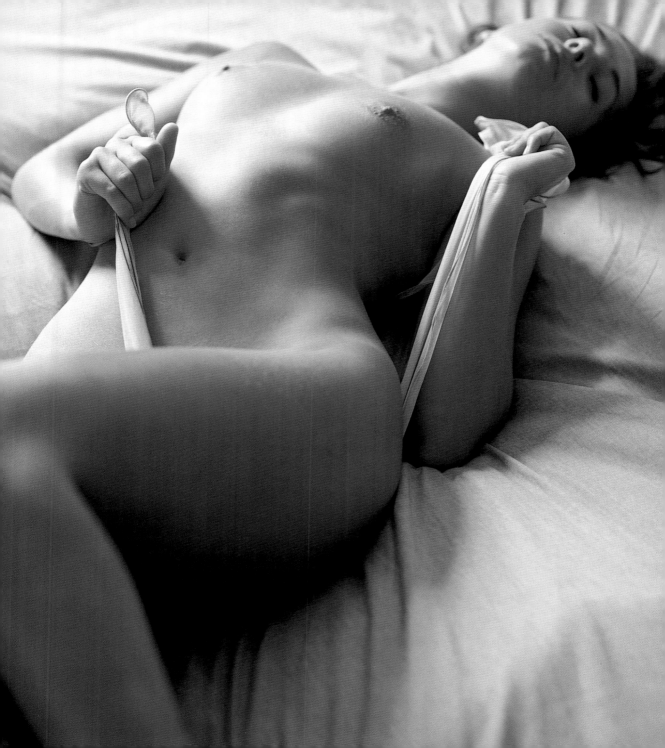

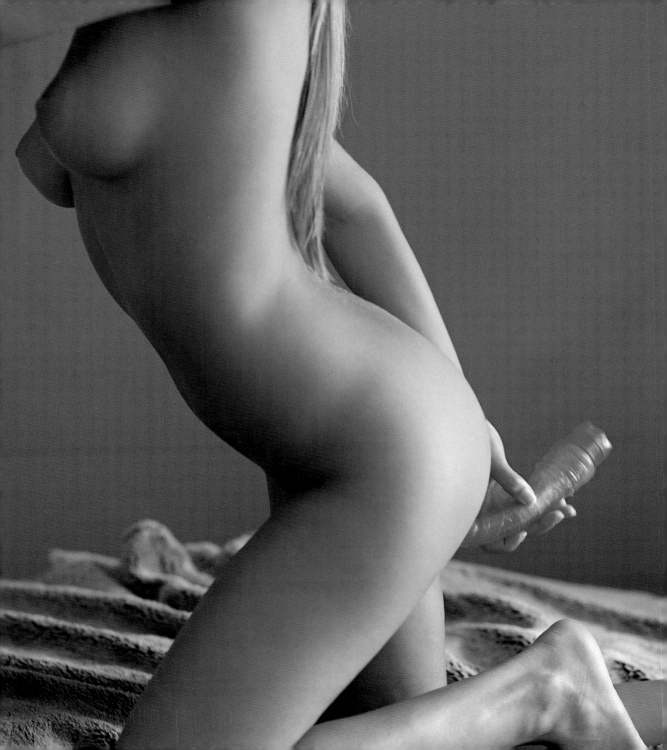

Going it alone

You can choose from an incredible range of vibrators and personal massagers, from the ever-popular Rabbit to G-spot vibrators, anal toys, love beads and stylish glass dildos that will burn a hole in your wallet. Experiment and discover what works for you.

The spice of life

Variety is key to pleasure. Most women find that they orgasm easily with a vibrator because the stimulation is steady and strong and, unlike your hand, a toy never gets tired. However, it's important not to rely too much on your plastic friend. Use your hands from time to time or try different forms of stimulation, like a pillow or a silk scarf. This will keep you tuned in to your body and you'll work out what does and doesn't feel good.

Keep it fresh

Go on, have fun with yourself – collect your own toy box, try water games in the shower or test out a vibrator designed for G-spot play. It's good to experiment a little and there are lots of innovative sex toys out there devoted to your pleasure (see page 52). Play with yourself at different times of the day and in a range of places. There's something decadent about having a little fun in the middle of the day in the office restroom.

Explore your body

Don't fall into the trap of having an orgasm in the same way every time: If it only takes a couple of minutes with a vibrator, solo play can become routine. Once in a while, try locking the doors, switching off your phone, burning some sensual aromatherapy oils and devoting yourself to your own pleasure. Enjoy a long bath, reconnect with your body and touch yourself all over. Take a proper look at your genitals using a mirror – what do they look like? How do they change when you touch them? Use a good lubricant to make the whole experience feel a lot more sensual. Look at your naked body in the mirror and remind yourself that you are gorgeous!

Feed your brain

Orgasms aren't just about the physical – your brain needs stimulation too. Read some erotica, listen to sexy music, watch good porn, lie back and let your imagination and hands wander. You'll find that orgasm comes more easily when you're turned on upstairs.

Clitoral pleasures

Despite Freud's insistence that clitoral orgasms are inferior to vaginal orgasms, it is now accepted by sexologists that the clitoris is, in fact, the most important organ for a woman's sexual pleasure. Extending some 9 inches inside the vagina, it is much larger than was previously thought. It contains 8,000 nerve endings – twice the number in the penis – and exists for pleasure-giving alone.

The science bit

Your clitoris is made up of different parts: the head, which sits under the clitoral hood at the top of the vaginal lips; the shaft; and two tips, which run along the vaginal lips internally. The only part you can see is the head, and this can be tricky to spot as its size and shape vary. What's important is the sensation it gives, and you can identify those spots where touch feels best. Using a water-based lubricant, gently push the hood back with your hand so you can see the head. Try different strokes and vary the pressure to find out what feels good. The head is extremely sensitive, so you might find it more pleasurable to focus on the surrounding area rather than directly on the head itself.

Close your eyes, use plenty of lubricant and fantasize…

Clitoral massage

The easiest and quickest way to have a clitoral orgasm is with a vibrator, but it's difficult to work out exactly what gets you going if you always rely on a toy. Here's how to give yourself a satisfying clitoral massage by hand.

Apply some lubricant and start out gently, using your thumb and index finger on the clitoral shaft. Slide the loose skin over the head back and forth so you can feel the shape of the head underneath. Try to work out how big it is. Move your fingers in circles and up and down until you discover what you like best, stimulating the head directly if it's not too sensitive, or the surrounding area if it is.

Once you start getting excited, increase the pressure and speed. If you have an orgasm, switch to a light stroke and leave the clitoris alone for a minute because it will be too sensitive to touch directly. Go back and stimulate it again if you want another orgasm. Take your time – it might take half an hour for you to orgasm, but it'll be worth it.

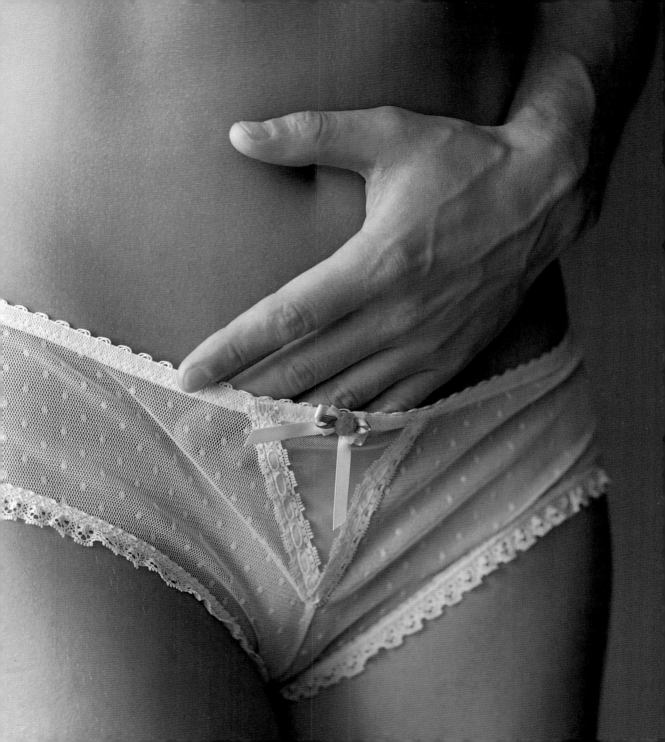

The G-spot mystery

There is much debate over the existence of the G-spot. Some women say they most definitely have one and that G-spot orgasms are much more intense than clitoral ones. For other women, the G-spot remains a mystery that they have long given up trying to uncover.

Grafenberg spot

The G-spot is named after Dr. Ernst Grafenberg, who discovered it in 1950. He identified a swollen spot near the top of the vagina, which apparently caused a woman to "ejaculate" during orgasm (see page 81). His theory remained unproven, however, and did not garner much interest until sex researchers Dr. Beverly Whipple and Dr. John Perry published a book on the subject in 1981, called *The G-Spot: And Other Recent Discoveries About Human Sexuality*. This book popularized the theory that women might be able to ejaculate and led to a public sensation.

The G-spot debate continues to this day. The latest thinking is that it is actually part of the clitoris, which researchers believe is much bigger than was previously imagined (see page 30).

So where is it?

Whatever the theory, if you haven't found yours yet, take a little time out to explore now. The G-spot is located a short way inside the vagina, on the front wall, behind your pubic area. It's quite tricky to find if you're lying on your back so try squatting. Insert two lubricated fingers inside your vagina so that they are slightly bent in a "come hither" motion, following your natural curve. It might help to play with yourself a little first so that you are aroused and to avoid irritating your bladder. You will feel a raised area, bumpy or ridged and a bit like a walnut. Congratulations – you've found your G-spot!

What now?

Applying direct, firm pressure, massage the area and keep going until it starts to feel good. Touching your G-spot may make you feel the need to pee, because you're pressing on the urethra, but this will go away. Some women report that they ejaculate and say a G-spot orgasm feels amazing, more like a whole-body orgasm than one that's focused on the genitals. (See page 81 for more on the G-spot orgasm and how to achieve it.)

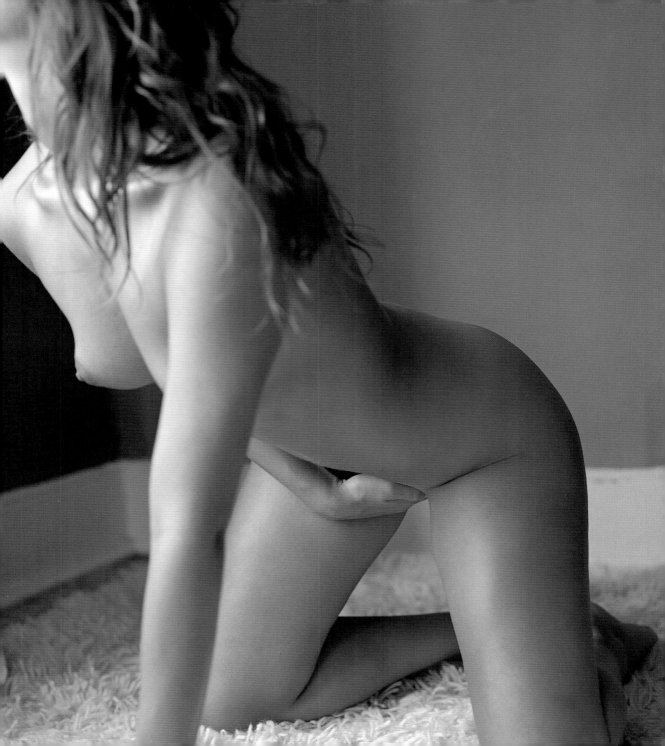

All about foreplay

Most women need plenty of foreplay and often complain they just don't get enough! This is because it takes us girls longer to orgasm than it does our men. For them, orgasm usually follows an erection; for us, a little more stimulation is required.

Take your time

Good foreplay can make sex seem more like a four-course meal than a hearty main course. Done well, it is an indication that your man cares as much about your pleasure and fulfillment as he does his own satisfaction. There's no denying that, sometimes, a quickie is just what we need but, if you've got the time, why not make more of sex?

Raise the temperature

First and foremost, foreplay is about the two of you. Think about what gets you both excited. Send each other sexy text messages or e-mails during the day, describing what you're going to do to each other later on. Create the right ambience with scented candles, music, aromatherapy, lighting, cushions – whatever raises the heat. Read or listen to erotica or watch some good porn together. Cook a sensual meal in the evening and feed tidbits to each other – a little champagne always helps!

Dress to undress

Wear sexy clothes that make you feel totally desirable and compliment your partner on what he's wearing. Dress in something that you know gets him going, and then take it off. Perform a striptease or a little erotic dance for him (see pages 64–67). The way you undress and touch yourself can make a big difference; let your partner know that you want to spend a little time getting ready for sex. Take a shower or bath together – and look but don't touch!

Kiss yourselves senseless

Once you are naked, start with an erotic body massage (see page 69) to really get you in the mood. Let him know when he does something that drives you wild. Research has shown that a woman's number one hot spot is her lips. There is a direct link from these to the clitoris and you will feel a good kiss in your entire body. Have a kissing session for at least 20 minutes. Kiss each other on the lips, neck, arms, thighs, tummy – everywhere except the genitals.

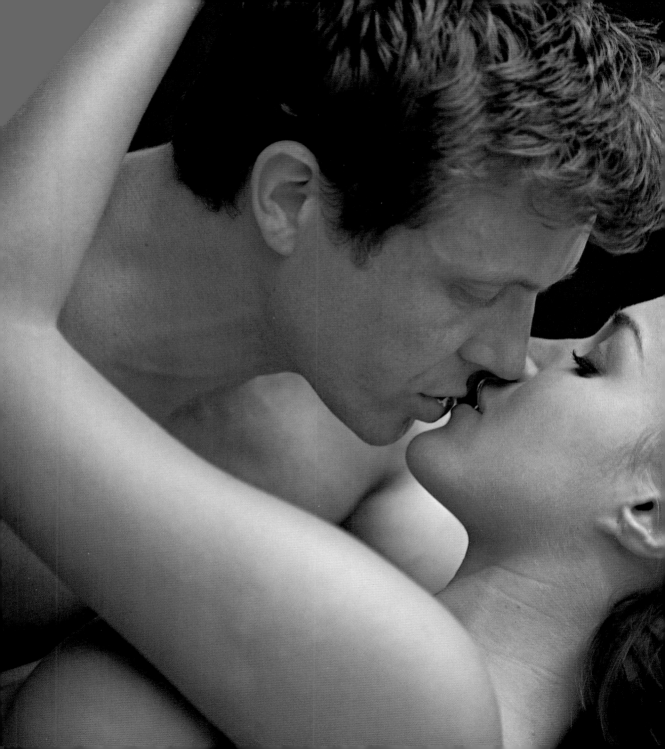

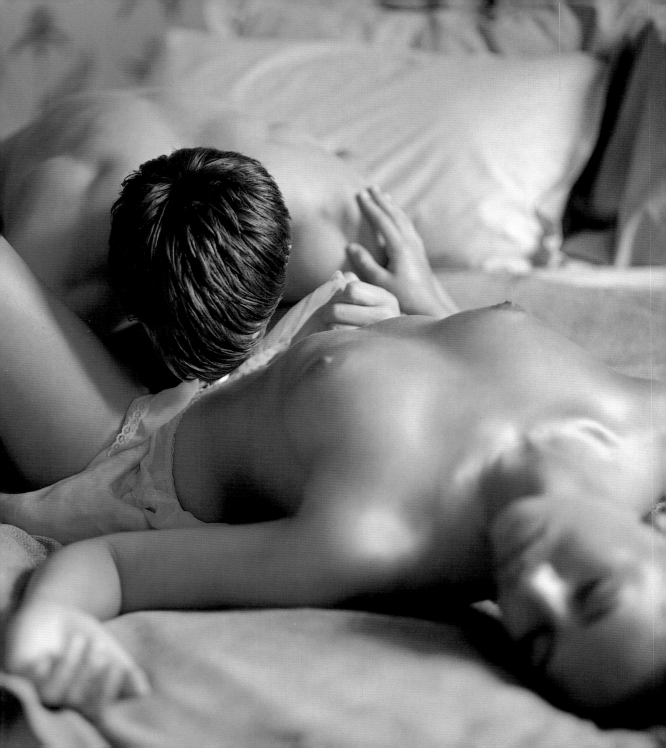

Oral tips for your man

- **Get him to tease you first.** He should kiss your tummy, thighs and buttocks before moving to your genitals. Make sure you're relaxed and have plenty of time – this isn't a rush job.
- **Ask him to start out slow.** He should lick your vagina from top to bottom and vice versa; circle your lips; go back and forth, up and down until he works out what you like. Tell him to vary the pressure and stroke to keep you guessing.
- **Focus on the clitoris.** Ask him to suck and tug on it very gently. Tell him what you like.
- **Finger play is good.** While he is licking your clitoris, suggest he inserts two fingers into your vagina. He could use his tongue to penetrate you, too.
- **Get him to suck a mint or ice cube.** Sucking on something cold while he licks you can feel sensational. A little whipped cream can be fun too.
- **He could try humming gently** – you'll feel the vibrations in your clitoris!

Cunnilingus

Most women just love receiving oral sex, both as foreplay and as an easy way to orgasm. This is because the tongue is the strongest muscle in the body. It is also wet and highly versatile, unlike the penis, so a little tongue play can feel simply amazing.

Feeling awkward?

Let's face it, oral sex is a very intimate act and you are not alone if you feel a little shy about asking for it. Maybe you are worried about how you smell and taste down there? Don't be – he'll love it – but if you are feeling paranoid, take a shower together beforehand. Drinking plenty of pineapple juice during the day will make you taste sweeter down below. If either of you is worried about hygiene or safety, use a dental dam (see page 86). Once past your inhibitions, you will find oral sex a great intimacy builder, because you expose yourself in front of your partner and it's a great way to really get to know each other's bodies – juices and all!

Fellatio

It will come as no surprise to learn that most men adore receiving oral sex – your mouth feels just like a hot, moist, super-flexible vagina! This is wonderful foreplay, so make time for it and be enthusiastic in the knowledge that you are giving him exquisite pleasure.

Try something different

It's easy to feel daunted about what technique to use, so find out what he likes first. Don't just use your mouth, but your fingers too. Stimulate his thighs, then move on to his shaft, testicles, scrotum, perineum and his prostate gland, which is a small gland hidden in the rectal area (see page 102). To find it, gently rub his anus or slip your finger inside (make sure your nails are short and your finger is well lubricated). If you do this at the same time as you play with his penis, your man will be in heaven – no doubt about it.

Most importantly, you should try to enjoy the experience yourself – he'll know if you're bored or half-asleep. If you're worried about health risks, use a flavored condom.

On this page are some tips for spicing up your oral technique, whether you use it as foreplay or to bring your man to orgasm. For a blow-by-blow account of giving the killer blow job, turn to page 101 in the section on male orgasms.

Oral tips for you

- **Start by teasing him.** Kiss the area around his penis – his inner thighs, buttocks, tummy, testicles – slowly making your way towards his penis. The glans is the most sensitive spot, and licking the frenulum (the ridged bit beneath the glans) will drive him wild.
- **Go deep.** Men love deepthroating – when you take as much of his penis as possible into your mouth. You'll probably gag if he starts thrusting, so ask him not to. Get around this by taking his penis into the side of your cheek rather than your throat or by making sure you're positioned so that your mouth and his shaft are aligned.
- **Try lubricant.** Rub lubricant or even whipped cream over his shaft for an extra erotic touch.
- **Use sex toys.** A vibrator on his penis or a vibrating cock ring will feel fabulous.

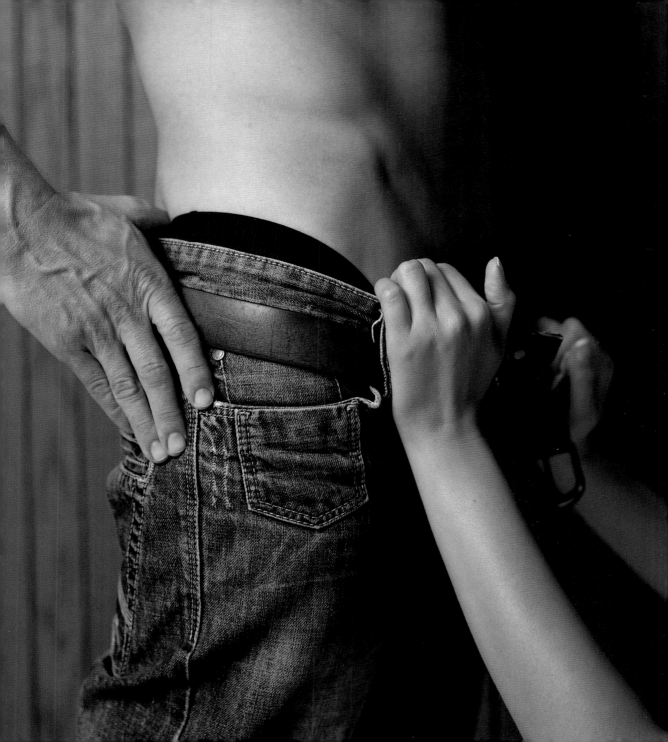

Tantric genital massage

A great way of giving and receiving pleasure, a Tantric genital massage makes brilliant foreplay. It can also help to intensify your orgasm and is good for working through any sexual blocks or problems. The female version is known as yoni massage, and the male as lingam massage. (*Yoni* is the Sanskrit word for vagina, and *lingam* is the word for penis.) A Tantric massage is fantastic for maintaining physical contact and intimacy – especially if you don't want to have full sex.

Yoni massage

Create a sensual atmosphere with fabrics, lighting, candles, music and aromas. Make sure the room is warm enough for you both to be naked. When you are ready, lie down on your back with pillows under your head. Put a pillow under your hips and spread your legs slightly so that your vagina is exposed. Start the massage by taking a few deep breaths and connecting with each other.

Your partner should start to relax you by gently massaging your legs, tummy, thighs and breasts. With his hands over your vagina, he can pour some water-based lubricant into one hand so it drips through to your vagina. Then he can gently massage your labia and mound, taking his time. He can squeeze the outer lip between his thumb and forefinger, sliding up and down and repeating on the inner lips. Gauging your reactions, he should vary the speed and pressure for maximum pleasure.

He should stroke your clitoris backwards and forwards, making small circles, squeezing and tugging on it gently. The point at this stage isn't to give you an orgasm but to relax your vagina.

Now he can insert his middle finger into your vagina to massage you internally. If you wish, he can make a "come-hither" motion to stimulate your G-spot (in Tantra, the sacred spot). Again, he should vary the speed and pressure, using the thumb on his right hand to stimulate your clitoris at the same time. If you have no objections, he could also stimulate you anally. He should use his other hand to massage your breasts or tummy. Keep breathing deeply as you approach orgasm. You may have more than one and, in Tantra, this is known as "riding the wave." Your partner should end the massage by slowly removing his hands and giving you a cuddle.

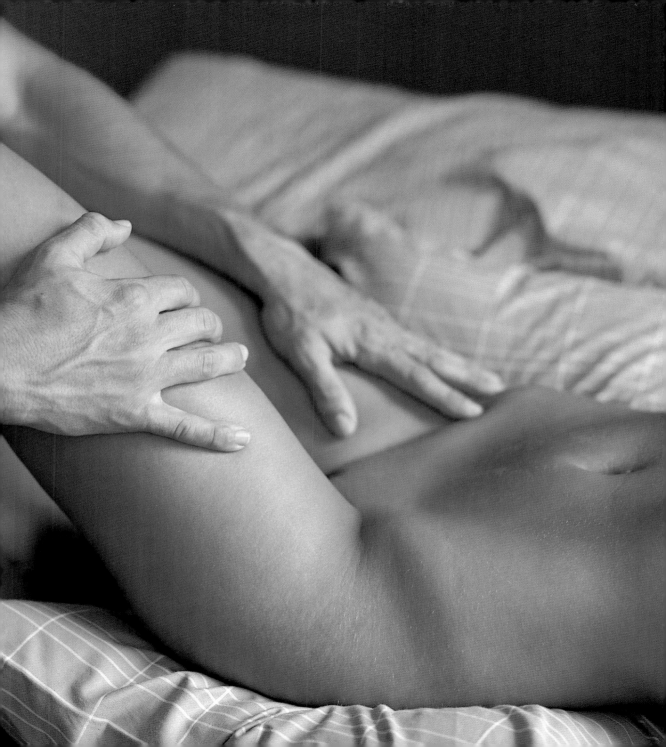

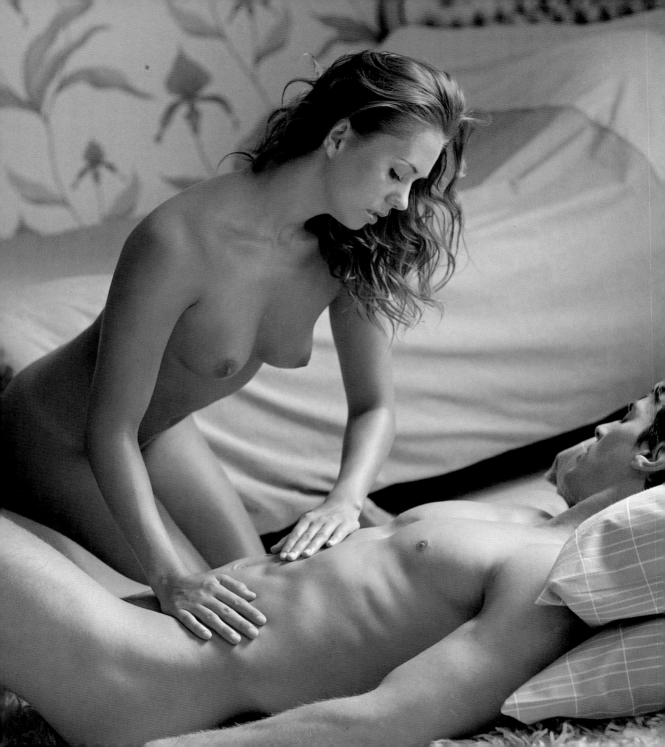

Lingam massage

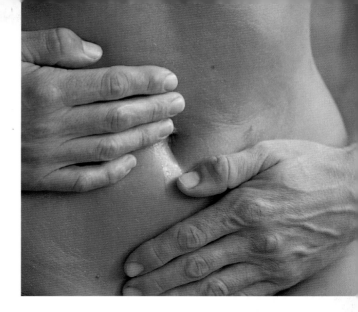

Lingam means "wand of light." In Tantric sex, the penis is seen as a conduit for creative energy and pleasure. The aim is to externally massage his penis, testicles, perineum (the pea-sized area between his testicles and anus) and his prostate area (sacred spot) so that he can relax and enjoy pleasure. If it is your man who usually initiates sex, a Tantric massage will allow him to let go and receive.

Ask your partner to lie down on his back, with pillows under his head so he can see you, and a pillow under his hips. He should spread his legs apart so that his knees are slightly bent and you can reach him easily. Start out with deep breathing to relax and focus you both.

Begin by gently massaging your partner's legs, tummy, thighs, chest and nipples. Pour some water-based lubricant into your hand so it drips through to his penis and testicles. Massage his scrotum,

His prostate – or sacred spot – is the male equivalent of the female G-spot

perineum and his anal area. Go slowly and vary the pressure. Try squeezing the base of his penis with your right hand, pulling up and off, and alternating hands so the motion is continuous. Change direction by starting at the glans of the penis and moving downwards.

Now massage the glans – it is highly sensitive and full of nerve endings. He might lose his erection and regain it, and this will feel great to him. If you sense he's about to come (his scrotum will tighten), stop massaging for a while. Doing this several times will strengthen his ejaculatory control. Tell him to breathe deeply to reduce his urge to come; once he's mastered this skill he'll be able to have sex for as long as he likes. Massage his sacred spot, pushing it inwards gently to make him feel it deep inside. Massage his penis with your right hand and his sacred spot with your left hand, pressing on this spot as he comes.

Sex games

You shouldn't take sex too seriously. Sexual play is all about awakening your senses and getting yourself in the mood. It allows you to experiment with your submissive or dominant side, and to discover new fantasies and turn-ons in the process. It's a very healthy way to explore your sexuality.

Where to start

There are a number of ways in which you can indulge yourself during the day and build up the sexual tension. Wear fabrics like cashmere, silk or satin that make you feel good and want to be touched. Drink a glass of red wine to get the blood flowing and help your muscles relax. Take a hot shower and really feel the water against your skin: This increases circulation and makes you more responsive to smell and touch. Make your home sensual with fabrics, cushions, lighting, flowers, music and aromas.

On the following pages you will find lots of suggestions for spicing up your sex life, from sex toys, kinky clothing and dirty talk to tips on living out your sexual fantasies, giving an erotic massage and putting on a special floorshow that will have him begging for more.

What does it for you?

- **Sexual fantasies.** Indulge in your wildest dreams, experimenting with different role-play situations. Read erotica, watch some porn, record yourself having sex.
- **Aphrodisiacs.** Find out which aromas and foods are a genuine turn-on for great sex.
- **Sex toys.** Enjoy new sensations and give each other pleasure in exciting ways.
- **All about lubricant.** Makes solo sex more fun and partner sex more enjoyable.
- **Lingerie.** Allows you to explore different roles in the bedroom.
- **Getting kinky.** Have fun with leather and rubber, whips and handcuffs.
- **Talking dirty.** Use naughty language to surprise and excite your partner.
- **Undress to impress.** Boost your sexual confidence and enhance your appreciation of your own body.
- **Erotic dance.** You'll love teasing him as you strut your stuff.
- **Erotic body massage.** A huge turn-on for both of you.
- **Mood enhancers.** Vices to spice up your sex life.

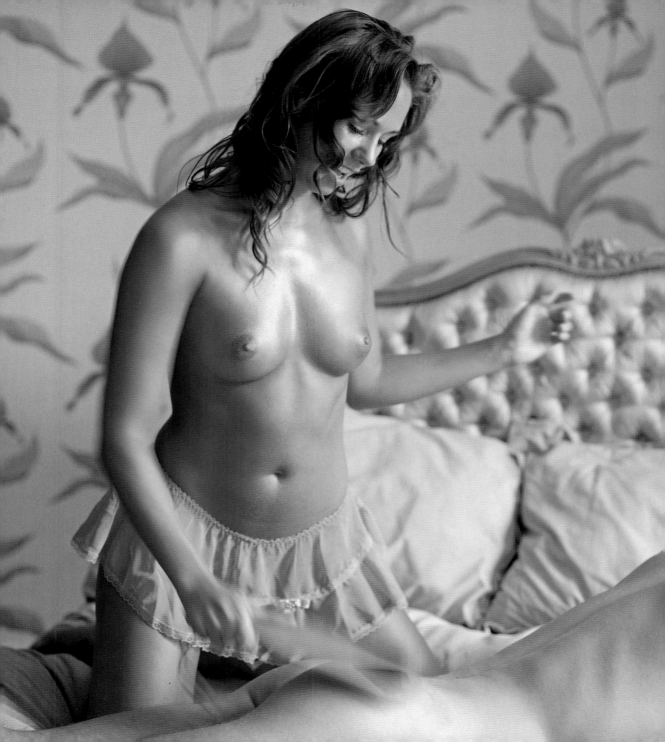

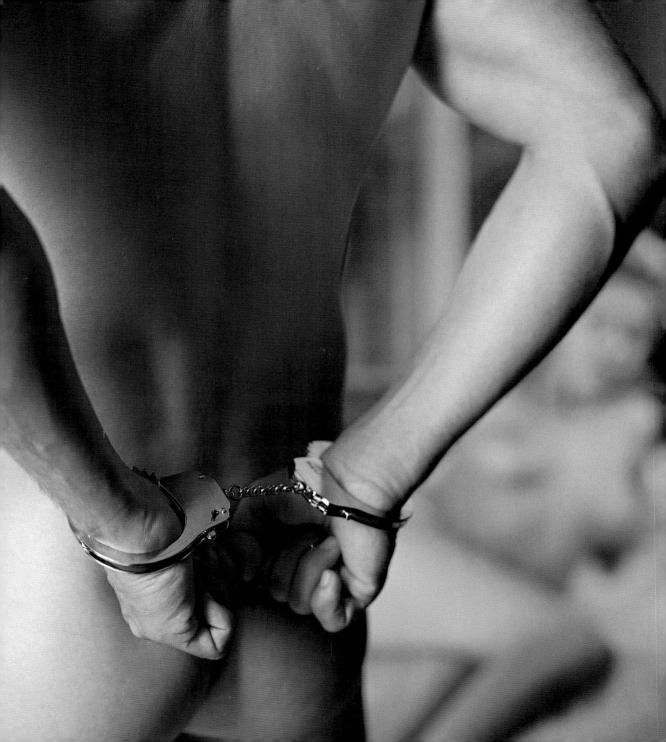

Sexual fantasies

Fantasies are an aphrodisiac, often because they put you in situations that are alien to you. You can use fantasies to explore your personality – if you are usually submissive, fantasize about being dominant – and you will probably learn something about yourself in the process.

Think what you like

Your fantasies may be so far removed from everyday life that you feel a little embarrassed even mentioning them to your partner. Having a dream about being taken by force doesn't mean that you want to be raped, however. Such fantasies are a completely normal way of expressing your sexual self, and they indicate sexual confidence and assertiveness in that you aren't simply waiting for someone else to turn you on.

Act it out

Share your fantasies with your partner if you want to, and use them to help spice up your sex life. Try role-play, dirty talk, or phone or internet sex with each other. If you are not sure where to start, keep a record of your sexual thoughts, read erotica or watch some female-directed porn.

e of the best

Having sex with someone else who isn't your partner – a celebrity, stranger or authority figure.

Being seen having sex or watching someone else have sex.

Being forced to have sex with one person or a group.

Sex with someone of the same sex.

Sex outdoors.

Double or triple penetration.

S&M or bondage activity.

Aphrodisiacs: aromas

Smell is the most powerful of the five senses, so much so that the smell of something that was familiar to you in childhood can transport you right back to a specific moment in your distant past. The scent of aromatherapy oils releases a range of neurotransmitters (chemicals) in the brain, which can transform your mood and create an immediate physical response in your body. For example, endorphins reduce pain and stimulate your sexual feelings, while serotonin relaxes you.

Using oils

Aromatherapy oils are highly versatile. You can use them in a burner to create atmosphere, in the bath or as massage oil. Certain oils, such as clary sage, jasmine, patchouli and ylang ylang will stimulate the pituitary gland, encouraging an interest in sex (this gland controls other glands, so a lack of interest in sex can result when it is inactive). In addition to these, oils that are considered aphrodisiacs include black pepper, ginger, fennel, frankincense, geranium, rose and sandalwood.

Boost your libido

Try the following combination in a burner:

- 2 drops of black pepper
- 2 drops of ginger
- 2 drops of sandalwood

Erotic massage

Add a few drops of one of the following to a base oil such as grapeseed or sweet almond:

- rose
- ylang ylang
- jasmine

Sensual bath

Try adding the following combination:

- 2 drops of rose
- 2 drops of patchouli
- 2 drops of ylang ylang

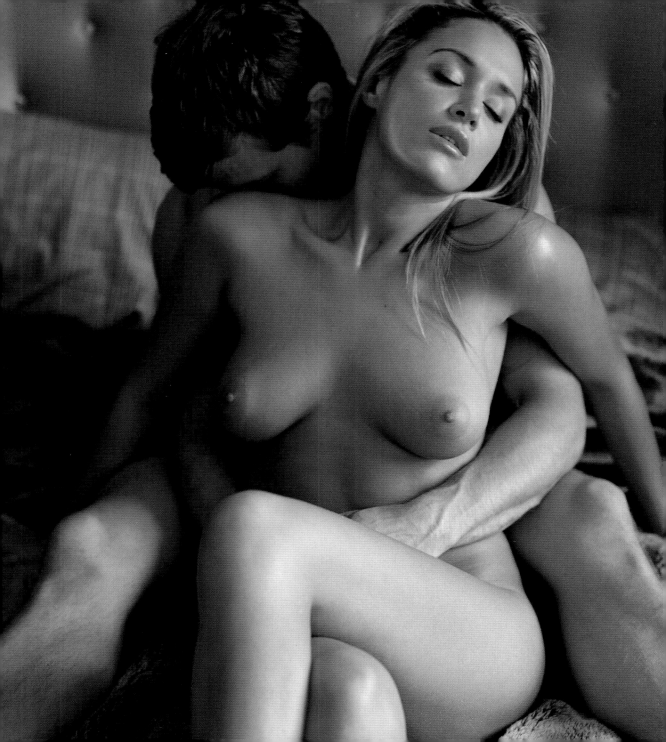

Aphrodisiacs: food

Food and sex have gone together as far back as Adam and Eve. Although there is no scientific evidence to prove that certain foods affect the libido, there definitely appears to be a psychological connection. The Romans, for example, believed that eating fruits and vegetables which resembled the genitals would make them sexually potent.

An orgasm diet?

American writer Marrena Lindberg has experimented with foods and devised an "orgasm diet," which she claims will increase your orgasm-ability. Having experienced problems with orgasms herself, she began using vaginal weight cones after pregnancy, to regain her pubococcygeus (PC) muscle tone. She also started taking fish oils as a supplement and found they increased her libido. After following her diet and exercise routine, she became able to achieve multiple consecutive vaginal and clitoral orgasms.

Want to give it a try? You will need to exercise your PC muscles regularly with a pelvic toner and consume fish oil, multivitamins and mineral supplements, as well as drink more juices – and eat dark chocolate!

Sensational foods

- **Caviar** enhances your nerve cells, supposedly making you feel more sexual.
- **Truffles** contain chemicals that are similar to a male sex hormone.
- **Chocolate** contains mood-improving stimulants. Good-quality dark chocolate seems to work best.
- **Coffee** drinkers are said to be more sexually active.
- **Spicy foods** such as garlic, curry, cumin and cayenne raise blood circulation and heart rate, making you feel horny.
- **Ginseng** increases the blood flow in your genitals and improves your libido.
- **Red wine** relaxes you and improves your blood flow.
- **Vanilla** smells delicious to men, who find it a real turn-on.
- **Mangoes** are considered sensual for their velvety texture and sweet, nectar-like juice.
- **Fresh figs** resemble a woman's genitalia.
- **Strawberries and whipped cream** can be used in all sorts of exciting ways.
- **Chocolate**, **jelly**, **honey** and **yogurt** are fun to smear on and then lick off!

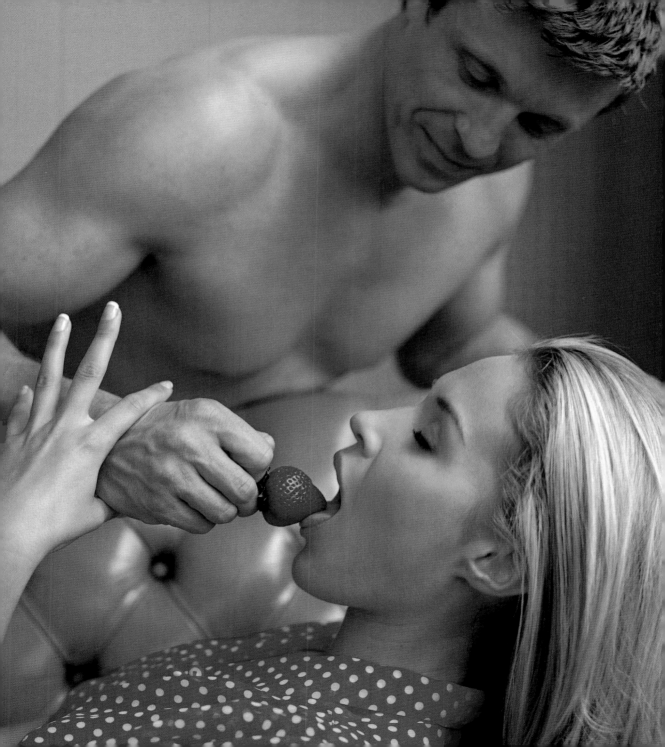

Sex toys for girls

Who doesn't enjoy sex toys? Most women learn how to orgasm using a vibrator; for some, this is the *only* way to orgasm. Ranging from cheap novelty to luxury, toys have been devised to serve your every need. What better way to spice things up in the bedroom? And there is no need to be embarrassed: With the help of the internet, your little indulgences couldn't be more discreet.

Vibrators

Made from silicone, latex, plastic jelly, rubber and glass, some vibrators look like penises, others more like tubes. Bestsellers include the Rabbit, based on the original Pearl Rabbit, which has a rotating shaft and G-spot "ears" for stimulating both the clitoris and the vagina. You can also buy vibrators for massaging the whole genital area or those that stimulate the G-spot directly.

Choose a finger vibrator for extra discretion or a strap-on one that leaves your hands free to roam elsewhere. Pay more for one made of silicone, which warms up to the temperature of your body, or experiment with a glass vibrator, adding to the sensation by heating it up or cooling it down.

Love eggs

Also known as egg vibrators or bullet vibrators, these are small egg-shaped vibrators that you insert vaginally. Most are made of rubber, metal, silicone or plastic. They are weighted and can be worn for longer periods to build up sexual tension. Some have an irregular rhythm to enhance your pleasure.

Finger vibrators

These are tiny vibrators that you slide onto the end of your finger for discreet clitoral stimulation. They are great for clitoral and vaginal lip stimulation and come with different-sized finger bands, so you can use them solo or with your partner.

Dildos

Non-vibrating sex toys come in all shapes and sizes. Dildos usually resemble a penis and can be used vaginally or anally, for solo sex or with a partner. The latest models are glass, which is not as flexible as silicone but can be warmed or cooled at whim, or "cyberskin," which is delicate and feels exactly like skin. You can buy double-ended dildos for dual penetration or harnesses with strap-ons.

Nipple clamps

Rubber-tipped clamps stimulate the nipples for extra sensation and to intensify orgasm. The clover clamp and the tweezer clamp both grip the nipple. Latest models vibrate and have various levels of pressure.

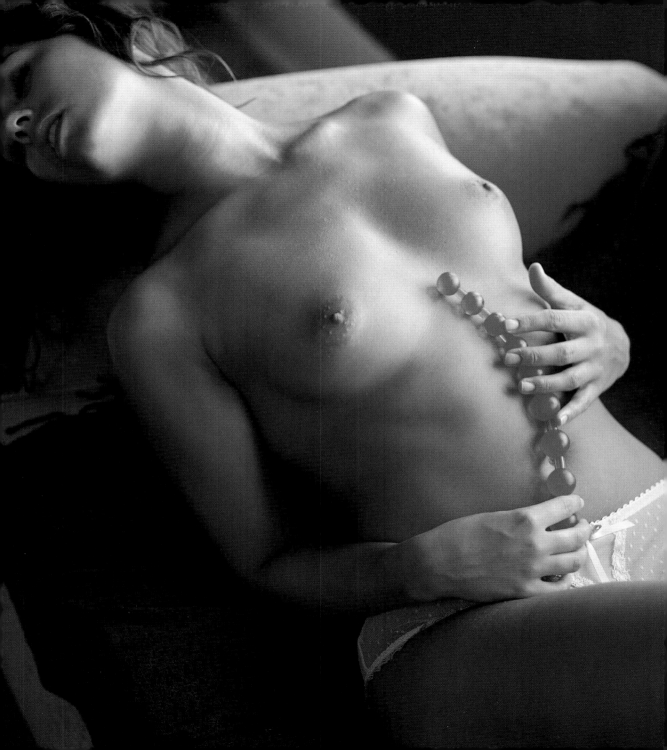

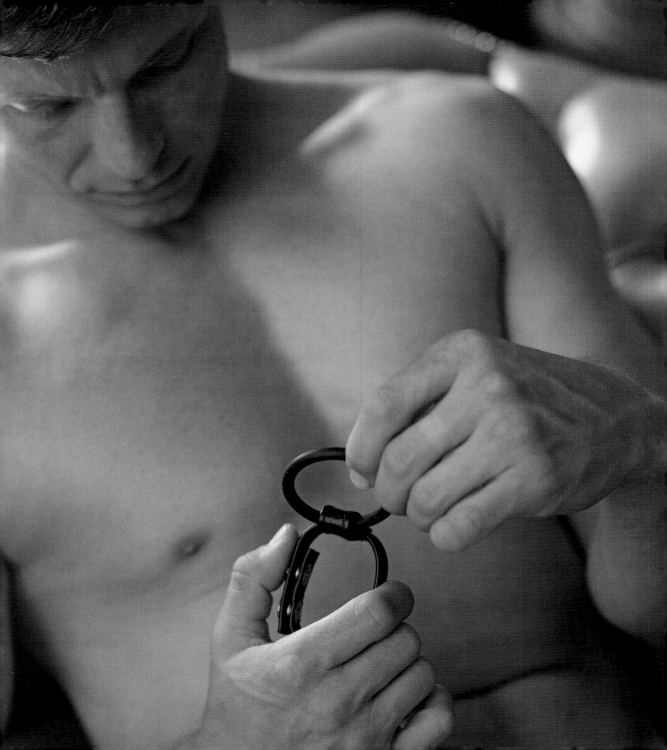

Sex toys for boys

Most men are a little shy when it comes to using toys, but once you've introduced your partner to a few, he will be raiding your toy box on a regular basis. Lots of men love having their nipples stimulated and are amazed by how good an anal toy feels since it directly stimulates the prostate gland. Using a vibrator on his penis while you give him oral sex can also vary the sensation for him and lessen the work for you.

Butt plugs

Similar to a dildo, a butt plug is smaller (and flared at the base so there's no chance of him losing it!). Men like them as they stimulate the prostate gland during sex. They come in all shapes and sizes; go for a smaller, thinner one if you've never used one before.

Prostate massagers

These anal toys stimulate the prostate. They look like thin vibrators and can be manual or non-manual. Non-manual types include the anal prostate-perineum massager, which gives intense non-ejaculatory orgasms, stimulating the two areas simultaneously. Manual types, which look more like a dildo with an angled tip, stimulate the prostate.

Cock rings

Designed to prolong an erection, cock rings sit around the base of the penis and testicles and squeeze the veins to keep blood trapped in the penis. It's also thought that they can delay orgasm.

There are various types, including vibrating ones and some that can tickle the clitoris during sex. Get a good fit and never leave it on for more than half an hour as this can cause nerve damage.

Penis pumps

These toys are supposed to inflate the penis to its maximum size by increasing blood flow and stretching tissues without impairing ability to have sex. Use carefully to avoid damage to ligaments.

Penis extensions

These are extension sleeves that are fitted over the top of the penis before sex to enhance girth and length. They come in various sizes.

Realistic vaginas

Also know as "pocket pussies" or "masturbators," these toys enable men to simulate sex alone. They are shaped as vaginas, anuses or just a hole to penetrate.

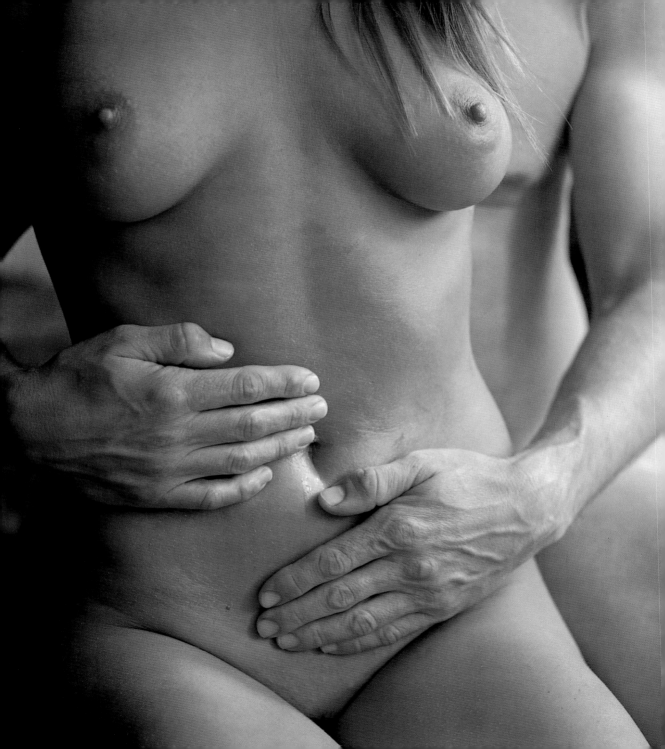

All about lubricant

You might think that you should be able to do the job yourself, but a good lubricant can definitely enhance your sex life. There will be times when you are dry down there: Hormones, periods, childbirth and breastfeeding all take their toll. Alcohol and drugs may also affect your ability to self-lubricate, as can stress, overwork and tiredness.

Why use lubricant?

Using lubricant makes solo sex more fun and partner sex more enjoyable. No matter how horny you feel, your vagina doesn't automatically lubricate. Lubricant also makes giving head a lot easier and it is essential for anal sex, as this part of the body doesn't lubricate itself naturally. Lubricants have come a long way: These days they can be flavored, made with natural ingredients, longer-lasting and non-sticky. Oil-based, water-based and silicone-based lubricants all have different properties.

Oil-based

Made from butter or vegetable oils, oil-based lubricants are great for massage, but avoid using scented ones for intimate areas – your genitals are sensitive and easily irritated. Vegetable or mineral oils are best: Coconut oil is very popular with men and smells great. You can use non-scented oils for masturbation, but don't use petroleum jelly as this will linger in your vagina for days. Bear in mind that oils destroy latex, making condoms ineffective. They can also damage toys containing latex.

Water-based

Made from water and glycerine, these are better for genital areas and good for intercourse because you can use them with condoms. They don't taste like anything and won't stain or irritate the body, plus they are easy to wash out. They dry out easily, however, and can become quite sticky (solved by adding water). Some men find that they reduce sensation and friction, and that they can't feel anything after a while. In this instance, wipe off with a damp cloth and start again.

Silicone-based

The crème de la crème of lubricants, these are sleek and oily, waterproof but non-greasy and can be used safely with condoms. They last longer, allowing you to stay slippery for ages. They also don't taste like anything. The only disadvantage is that they are more expensive and are harder to wash off (you'll need soap and water). It is best not to use them with your silicone toys because they can cause damage to items made from this material.

Lingerie

Lingerie *is* romance. Wearing fabulous underwear alters the way you feel about your body, making you walk taller and feel sexier. It can also have quite an effect on your foreplay: Men are visual creatures and they love to be seduced by flimsy fabrics that reveal more than they conceal. Turn yourselves on with something sensual and you will not fail to light his fire.

Indulge yourself

Choose whatever takes your fancy from the wide range of colors and fabrics available. Plain black or white are sexy classics, while pink and peachy colors look good on most skin tones. Go for the hot pinks and purples if you want to step up a gear. You can opt for stretchy fabrics to flatter your body shape and chiffon or lace for a romantic, baby-doll look. Dressing up in flimsy panties is always fun, and undressing even more so. Choose underwear that you want to show off and sex up the look with fun accessories like nipple tassels, boas, sequins, stockings and garters.

It is worth getting your bust size checked if you are buying new underwear; surveys have established that some 85 percent of women are wearing the wrong size of bra. Most department stores offer bra fittings. If you're looking for something extra-special (or your partner wants to treat you), try a bra fitting for a handmade item at a more exclusive boutique for a garment with a Parisian haute-couture touch.

Reinvent yourself

You can use lingerie as a way of developing your sexual style or creating a new persona in your sex repertoire – be it burlesque performer, striptease artist, dominatrix or baby doll. Add a new dimension to sex with peephole bras and crotchless panties – both of which are equally convenient for solo sex and initiating sex in different situations. The slightly naughty element will make you feel very sensual and especially aware of your body and physical sensations.

Your lingerie drawer

Classic items you should have for playtime include a corset, high heels, stockings and garters. Half the fun is wearing them: the rest is removing them and using them to seduce your partner. Once you're undressed, he's hardly likely to object if you use a pair of silk stockings to blindfold him while you remove his clothing, slowly but surely!

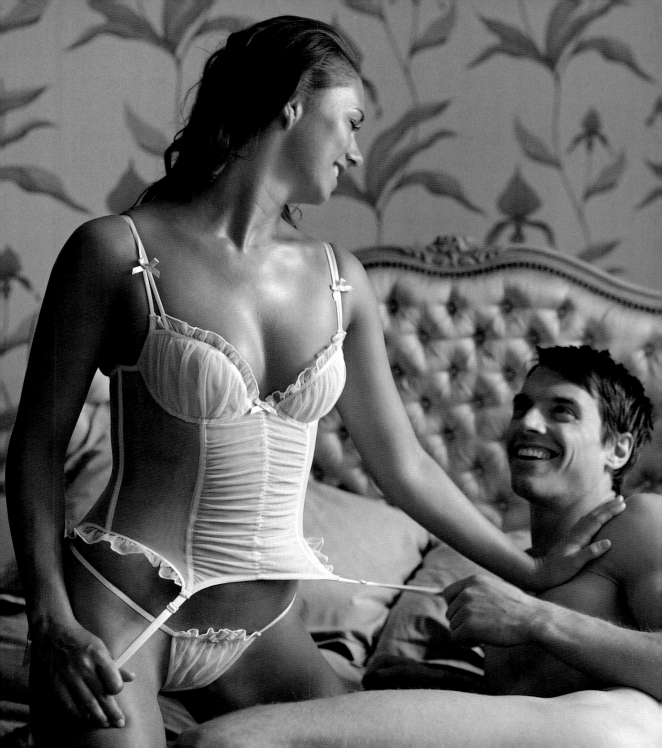

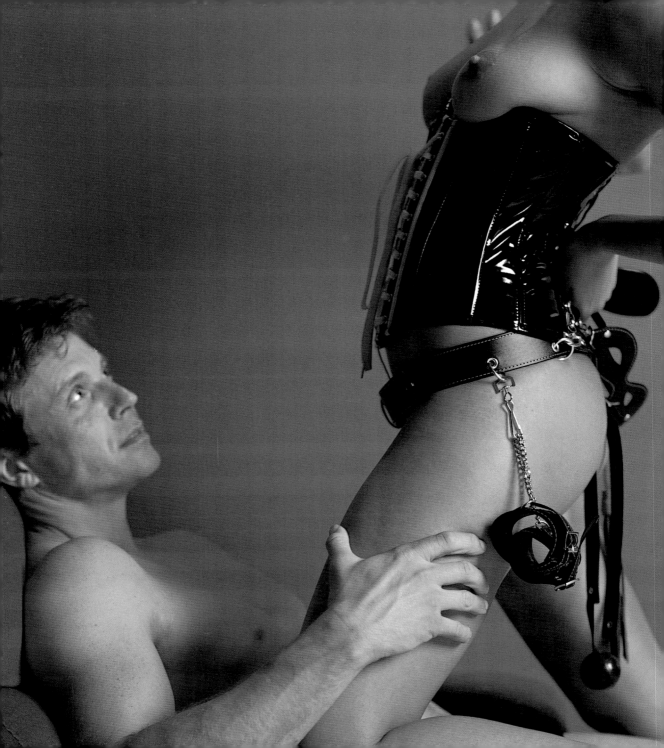

Getting kinky

Dressing up should be an integral part of sex play, allowing you and your partner to explore your wildest sexual fantasies. Donning a fantasy costume, whether it's as a nurse, dominatrix, secretary, biker or police officer, will allow you to explore your sexual identities and boost your sexual confidence to no end.

Try it out

Experiment with role-play scenarios and you'll probably find you have several fantasies about how you'd like each other to look. Work with your own accessories to start. You can buy or rent most of the classic costumes in standard dress shops, and it's worth checking out some of the female sex shops for original costumes and new ideas. The internet is also a great resource if you're a little shy or want to browse for ideas.

The right location

If the bedroom doesn't seem the right place for acting out your fantasies, try a new venue. If you have a secretary or teacher fetish, get a hotel room for the night and turn it into a boardroom or classroom. Buy some accessories such as canes, ties and gloves to complete the theme. Fetish clubs are also fabulous for exploring your costume fantasies in a safe environment and can provide a great source of inspiration.

Getting kinky is all about body confidence

What works best?

Rubber and leather both look and feel sexy because they are tight, but can be uncomfortable and hot to wear for long periods. Keep your leather outfits short and sweet and dust yourself in talcum powder first. A good alternative is PVC: It's lighter and cheaper, and there are a good range of fun outfits available. Don't fool yourself into thinking that you have to be model-skinny to wear leather and rubber outfits. There's nothing sexier than a curvy woman clad in leather.

Don't overlook the shoes – most men have a footwear fetish of one sort or another. Perhaps your man is turned on by the sight of you in a pair of stilettos, gets a thrill out of sucking painted toenails or loves the pleasure-pain feeling of your heel against his skin. There will be something, so make sure you have a pair of fuck-me shoes in your closet.

Talking dirty

It is easy to forget that your voice is just as important as dressing up or using a new toy when it comes to sex play. It may seem daunting at first, but talking dirty really can intensify sex. It's not about reciting lines from a porn movie or uttering the filthiest words you can think of; it's about using language to delight and surprise each other when you are least expecting it.

Still not convinced?

Sexy talk is all about making your partner feel like the most important and desired person in the world. Make aural seduction a part of your day. Whisper naughty things to each other in public or while you are at the office, and send dirty texts about what you plan to do later. Flatter each other. Point out the small things that you adore about each other. Tell him if he does something that makes you feel special or if you love an outfit he wears. Compliments boost our sexual confidence and make us feel good about ourselves.

Once you get into the bedroom, start by reading erotic stories to your partner. If that doesn't appeal – if you just know DH Lawrence isn't going to turn him on – write out a fantasy of your own and read it in bed. Encourage him to do the same and get into the habit of describing your fantasies in detail to each other. Speak slowly as you do so; it is more intimate and signals that you have all the time in the world for him.

And during sex?

The words you whisper into each other's ears or cry out during sex don't have to be x-rated. It's best to be natural and spontaneous and avoid rehearsing what you plan to say. If you feel sexy you'll sound like it, and letting go of your inhibitions will really turn your partner on.

Think of different words to describe your genitals or a sex act, and describe exactly what you plan to do. Tell your partner, with feeling, what you want him to do or ask him to tell you what he wants and how he'd like you to do it. If you feel self-conscious about expressing yourself vocally during sex, choose one word to explain what you want – like "harder" or "faster" – or groan and moan louder when he does something you like. And remember: There are different levels of dirty talk – soft and hard. Start out soft, using gentle phrases like "I want to feel you," and leave the saucier bits for later when you're both totally turned on.

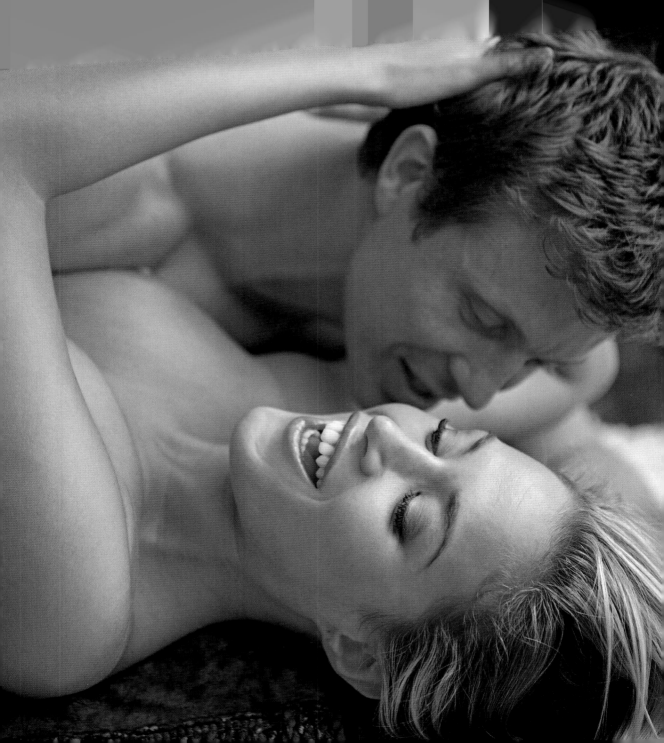

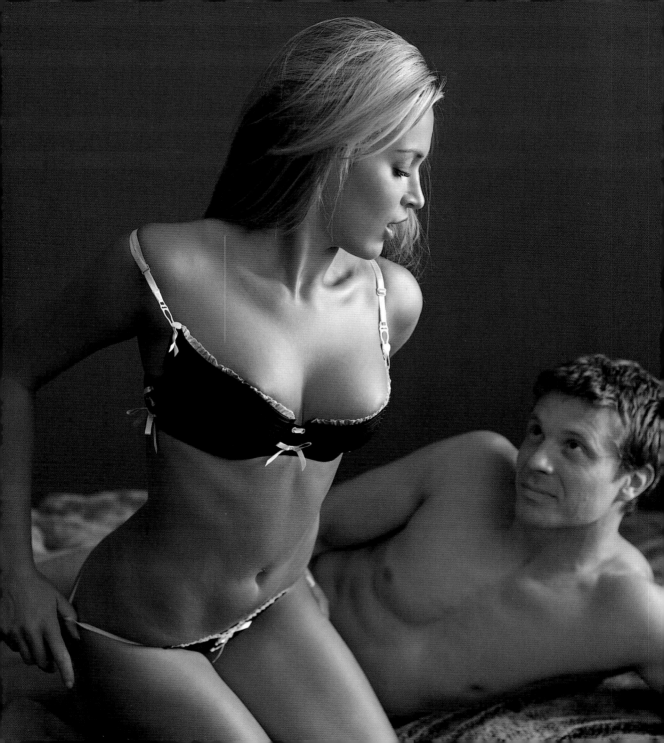

Undress to impress

Striptease is an ancient art that has been performed by various cultures for centuries. There are accounts in ancient mythology – including the infamous Dance of the Seven Veils of Salome – and variants are still practiced today in countless clubs and bars. Get into the mood and you'll find undressing for your partner is fun, stimulating and erotic. Remember that striptease is all about attitude and confidence – feel sexy and you'll be sexy!

Set the scene

Create the right ambience using candles or red light, and make sure you have enough space. Add fresh flowers, a chilled bottle of wine and some exotic nibbles. A large mirror will make the show even more exciting for him. Stripping takes a certain amount of physical and mental preparation – take your time and enjoy it. Have a scented bath. Shave, exfoliate and use good-quality body lotion. Give yourself a manicure and pedicure. Sip from a glass of that wine as you go.

What to wear

A good striptease is all about the layers – you need several so you can take them off slowly. You will tantalize your partner by never being completely naked. Nipple tassels or a G-string will offer the most minimal of cover. Use plenty of accessories: silk scarves, a feather boa, belts and a hat. Wear clothes that are easy to get out of, and have a

practice run beforehand so you feel confident. High heels will enhance your legs, but you also need to be able to walk in them! If you have a killer little black dress, wear that. Flaunt your best parts through your clothing: A chiffon or silk gown will cover you in a sensual way and enhance your curves.

Enjoy the show!

If you're nervous, blindfold your man when he comes in and whisper your intention in his ear. Strip to slow and sensual music, starting with small items – earrings and accessories – tossing them casually towards him or behind you. Gradually build the tension: Slip a strap off your shoulder, turn around and back again. The idea is to tease him until he can bear it no longer. Make full use of the room and enjoy it as much as he does. And if you have to abandon your routine midway because he can't keep his hands off you, it's been a success!

Erotic dance

Sexy dancing – using your whole body to simulate sex – is a variation on striptease and an excellent form of foreplay. Not only that, erotic dancing will boost your self-confidence, keep you fit and provide a truly visual treat for your partner. It will make you very aware of your body and posture and, with practice, you'll notice a real difference in the way you move and hold yourself.

Learn the moves

If you want to practice a routine at home, look for an erotic dance DVD that teaches the basic moves. Better still, take a class in your area or go to a lap-dancing club with your partner. This is an intimate treat and you'll probably find it just as much of a turn-on as he does. Pole-dancing is gorgeous to watch, but a lot harder than it looks. If you want to try it out, you can buy a pole for practicing simple, fun moves at home.

Follow your instincts

Get yourselves in the mood with a glass of wine before you start. Dim the lights for the right ambience – your fabulous body will look sexier too. Wear clothes and lingerie that feel good to touch. Sensual dance is as much about confidence and attitude as it is about fancy moves. Follow your basic instincts, moving slowly and wiggling your body as you go. Get into your curves!

Keep just out of reach and he'll find you totally irresistible

Walk the catwalk

Approach and withdraw from your lover, imagining that you're on a catwalk. Step forward slowly, keeping your eyes on him and using your hands to caress your body as you get nearer. As you dance, remind yourself that you are sexy. Touch yourself the way you'd like your partner to touch you. Roll your hips as you turn around and retreat. Then approach again, using your eyes to communicate with his. This time come closer, but take your time. Dancing is about sharing your body with your partner. Get close enough for him to sense your movements. Allow your hair to brush against his face, a hand to stroke his neck. It will feel exquisite to him and he won't be able to take any more.

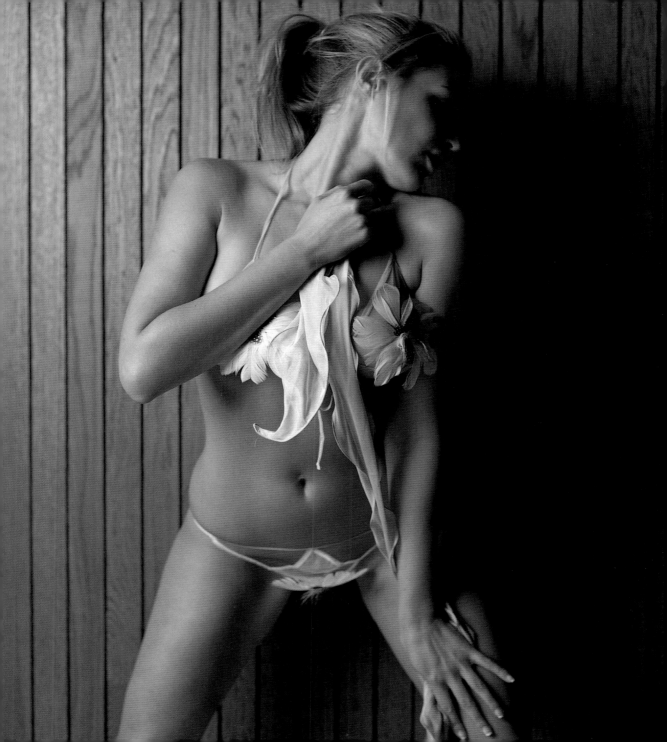

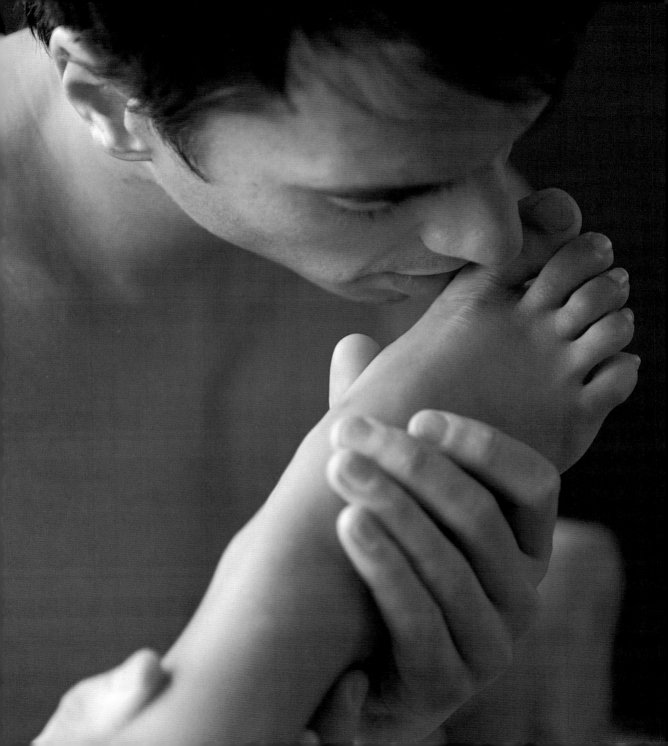

Erotic body massage

Giving an erotic body massage will boost your self-esteem, help you to view sex in a broader, more sensual way, and provide an intimate treat for your partner. Once you have worked on him, have him work on you (or vice versa). You can give the massage as a prelude to sex or as an act in itself. The most important thing is to take time to nurture each other's bodies.

Getting started

If you don't have a massage table, use a firm bed or a comfortable mat. Create your boudoir: Dim the lights and make the room warm and inviting. Use aromatherapy oils such as rose or jasmine to set the mood (see page 48). Turn off any phones so you won't be disturbed. Take a warm bath together so that you are both relaxed, and put on some calming music. Keep a towel handy for the parts you aren't massaging. Before starting, ask your partner if he would like you to massage his genitals (page 43 describes how to do a Tantric lingam massage).

The massage

With your partner lying on his stomach, work your way from top to bottom. Use a good lubricant or massage oil, warming it up in your hands before rubbing it into his skin. Start with his scalp, face and ears and move down to massage the neck, back, shoulders, arms, buttocks, legs, feet and toes.

Watch your partner's reactions to figure out what turns him on

Vary your stroke and ease out any knots that you find. We store tension in our buttocks; massaging here increases blood flow to the area and leads to better orgasms. Keep your movements fluid and constant. Kiss his body as you work – the skin is one big erogenous zone.

Get him to turn over, and repeat the process. There are more nerve endings on the front of the body, so he will be very responsive. Try sucking, gently pulling or pinching his nipples – it is possible for him to orgasm from nipple play alone (see page 107). Be creative to keep him feeling turned on.

A foot massage will relax his whole body. Hold a foot in one hand and massage the top with the other. Rotate each foot, massaging his ankles, toes, heels and bones. To finish, gently tug on his toes.

Mood enhancers

When you're stressed, busy and tired, your sex life is usually the first thing to suffer. Do not despair: There are plenty of ways to help your mind and body prepare for sex, including herbal supplements, sex-aid drugs and pheromones.

Herbal supplements

Herbal supplements such as damiana, ginseng and gingko biloba are well-known aphrodisiacs that can help us to feel more sexual. If you are suffering from a low libido, try damiana or dong quai, both of which promote hormonal balance. Your man can try saw palmetto, pygeum, stinging nettle or yohimbine, all of which aid the functioning of the male reproductive system, particularly the prostate gland. Ask a qualified herbalist for advice.

Drugs

The race is on to develop a female Viagra to increase sexual arousal in women. This project hasn't been successful so far because the female sexual response cycle is so different from that of the male, and what works for your man won't work for you. One drug currently in development is PT-141, touted as the "desire drug." It comes in the form of a nasal spray and is thought to work instantly. So far, studies on female rats have shown that it makes them pretty horny towards their male companions. If trials on humans go well, a new drug could be with us very soon.

Scentuelle

Simply smelling this clear patch, which emits multiple aromas, is supposed to boost desire levels, as the smell molecules affect brain activity. Wear it in an easily accessible place and sniff once an hour.

Pheromone perfumes

Perfumes containing pheromones are supposed to make us attractive to the opposite sex. This seems to be borne out of a 2002 study at San Francisco State University, which found that 74 percent of women wearing pheromone perfume experienced a 50 percent increase in male sexual attention, in the form of kissing, more dates and more sex.

Orgasmatron

American pain specialist Dr. Stuart Meloy initially invented this device to help women with chronic back pain; a surprising side effect was that it gave them orgasmic pleasure! A remote-controlled electrode inserted in the spine helps women with spinal injuries, back pain and nerve damage to experience orgasm. It's currently expensive, but Meloy is researching ways of making it cheaper.

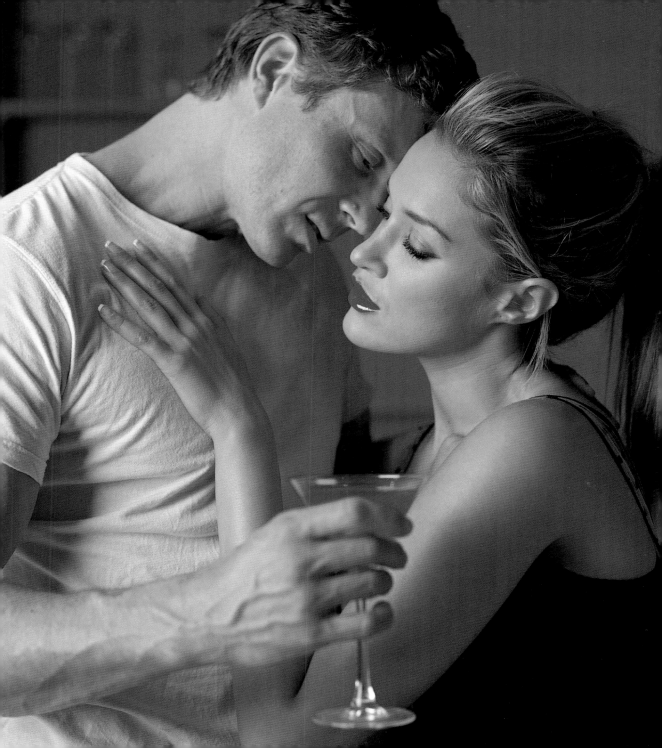

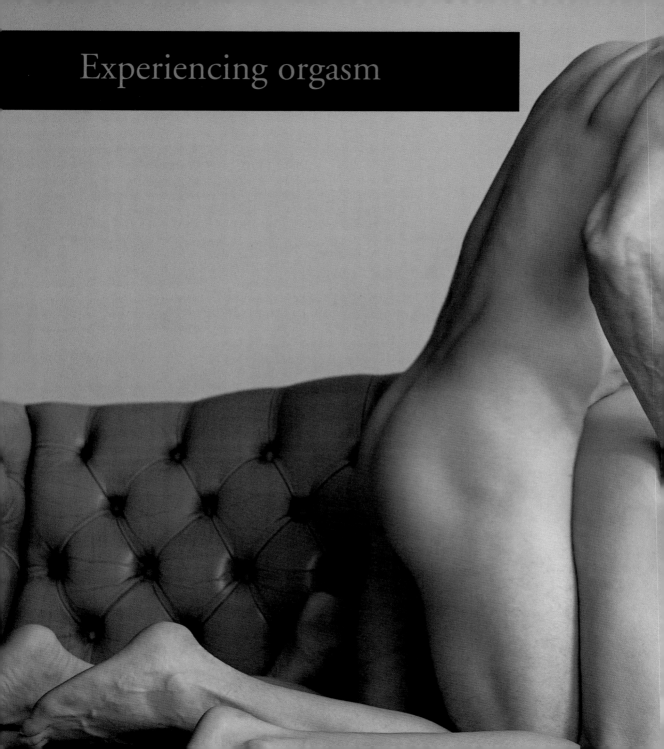

Experiencing orgasm

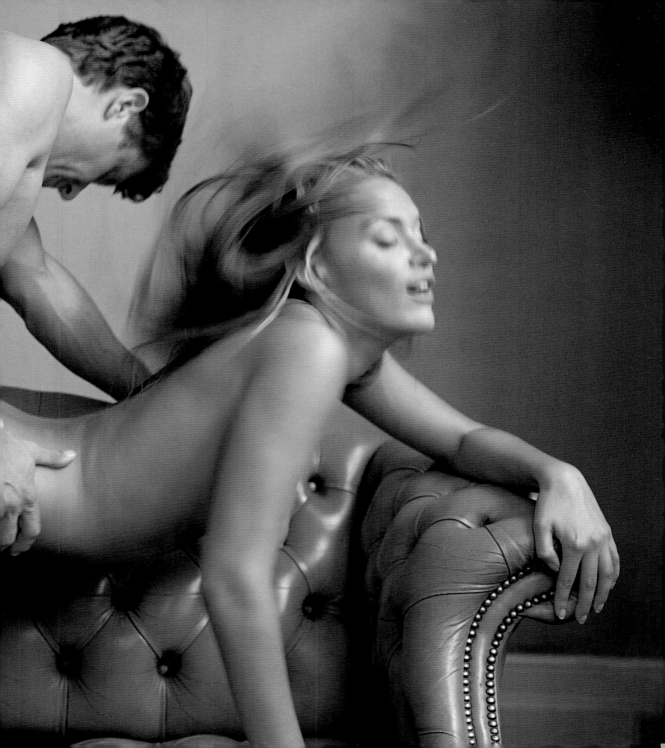

Way to go!

You have heard of the multiple and clitoral, but how about the fantasy orgasm – no genital stimulation required – or the nipple orgasm? If you take the time to explore your body, you'll find that it's full of unexpected erogenous zones. Orgasms are a state of mind and there are many things you can do to make them bigger and better.

Who said it was easy?

Changing attitudes have done much for the orgasm. It is no longer thought that the only time a woman should orgasm is at the same time as her partner, an attitude that was quite the fashion in the 1960s. While there is nothing wrong with the idea of simultaneous orgasm, it's something that can be hard to achieve (the trick is good foreplay and lots of it). For a woman, ability to orgasm in a certain way can also depend on where she is in her menstrual cycle, how much she's had to drink and even her general mood.

It's possible to have an extended massive orgasm – lasting up to three hours!

Room for improvement?

Luckily, we now know that there are many different types of orgasm, and some are much easier to reach than others. This section explores all the different orgasms that men and women can have and explains exactly how to have them. It covers the most common climaxes – clitoral, G-spot, vaginal – and also looks at a few less obvious ones, such as fantasy, anal and chest orgasms, and even a three-hour extended massive orgasm, as explored by sexperts Steve and Vera Bodansky. And since there's much to learn from the East when it comes to sexual pleasure, this section also describes some of the most orgasmic positions from the *Kama Sutra*, Tantric and Tao sexual traditions. The Eastern sexual traditions don't place as much emphasis on orgasm as a goal of sex; instead, sex is seen as a spiritual, whole-body encounter – an attitude from which we in the West can learn a lot.

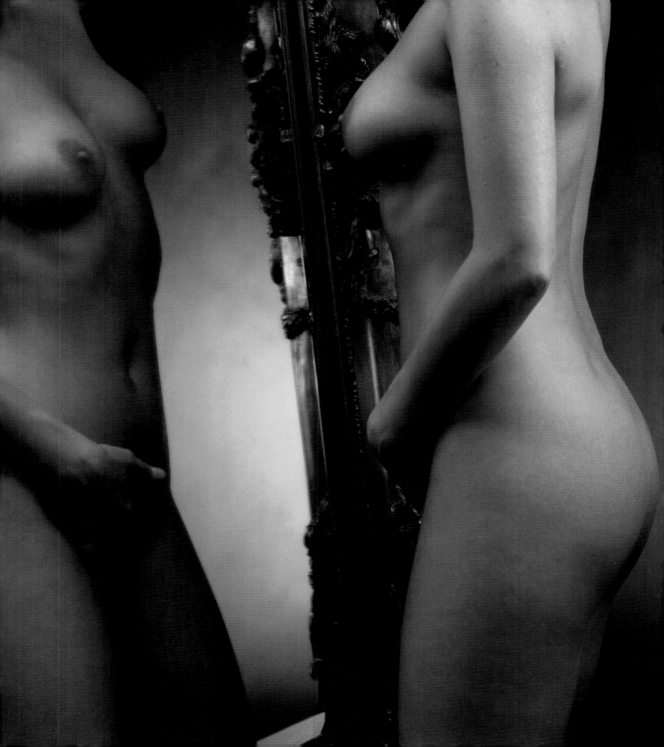

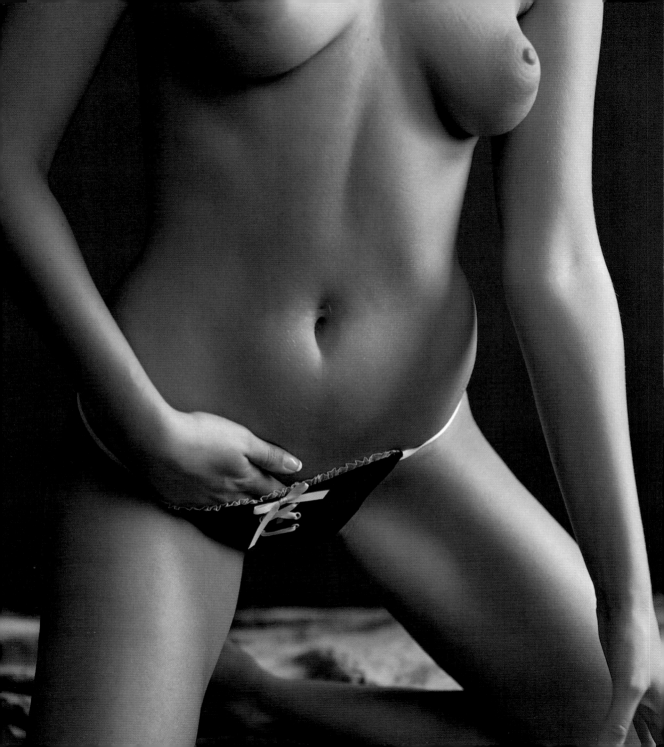

Your orgasms: clitoral

Clitoral orgasms are the most common type of climax and, usually, the most intense. The clitoris is a marvelous organ: It extends far back into the body and clitoral orgasms play over the whole of the highly sensitive pudendal nerve system. When the clitoris is stimulated to the max, you will feel the orgasm right across your vulval region – in your labia, clitoris, urethra and vagina.

Manual play

Ask your partner to put his hand on your pubis mons (the area above your pubic bone), with his fingers angled towards your clitoris. He needs to use plenty of lubricant and move his hand back and forth, or in circles, until he finds a rhythm you like.

You on top

When you're turned on and in the mood for sex, climb on top of your partner and guide his penis inside you. Being on top gives you control of stimulation to the clitoral area and you will be freer to move around to give yourself maximum pleasure. As you approach orgasm, tell your partner to start thrusting. Timing and practice are key.

The function of the clitoris is simply to give a girl pleasure!

Him on top

A popular variant of the missionary position is the coital alignment technique (CAT), which allows your partner to maintain contact with your clitoris while his penis is inside you. To do this, he needs to be positioned slightly higher up your body, so that his shoulders are above yours. He should penetrate you shallowly, using the base of his penis to stimulate the clitoral area as he thrusts. The combination of these two movements can give you an intense clitoral climax.

Need some help?

If he can't manage this for long without getting tired, try using a small vibrator on your clitoris, or stimulate it by hand, while he's inside you. And experiment with movement – you might find that you prefer side-to-side motions over up and down.

Your orgasms: vaginal

Vaginal orgasms are often described as a more all-encompassing experience than clitoral climaxes because you feel them in more parts of your body. Vaginal orgasms involve a different nerve system (the pelvic and hypogastric system) and affect your cervix and uterus as well as the genital area. There's also a difference in sensation. With clitoral orgasms, the uterus lifts up and back into the body, while with vaginal climaxes the uterus bears down. Vaginal orgasms are less common than the clitoral type, and are usually harder to reach.

You on top

Get on top during intercourse and move in a circular motion as your partner thrusts, stimulating both the clitoris and the vaginal area. This is a good position to try if you want deeper penetration and it allows you to control the thrusting and pressure. To vary things, face your partner's feet instead of his head. This frees you up to move in different ways and creates new sensations. The added mental stimulation of trying a new position will also make it that much more exciting.

You need to be pretty turned on to have one of these

Him on top

Have sex in the missionary position and try putting a pillow under your hips to elevate you. You can also raise your knees and tuck them into your chest. This will allow him to penetrate you deeply and you will feel him brush against your cervix each time he thrusts. It's thought that adopting this position can help you to conceive since it raises the cervix – helping the sperm to swim upwards! If you are hoping to get pregnant, lie flat on your back and don't move for half-an-hour after your orgasm. (And who's going to argue with that?)

Need some help?

Try using a bigger vibrator during masturbation, and do some work on your pubococcygeus (PC) muscles. Strengthening these will intensify your orgasms.

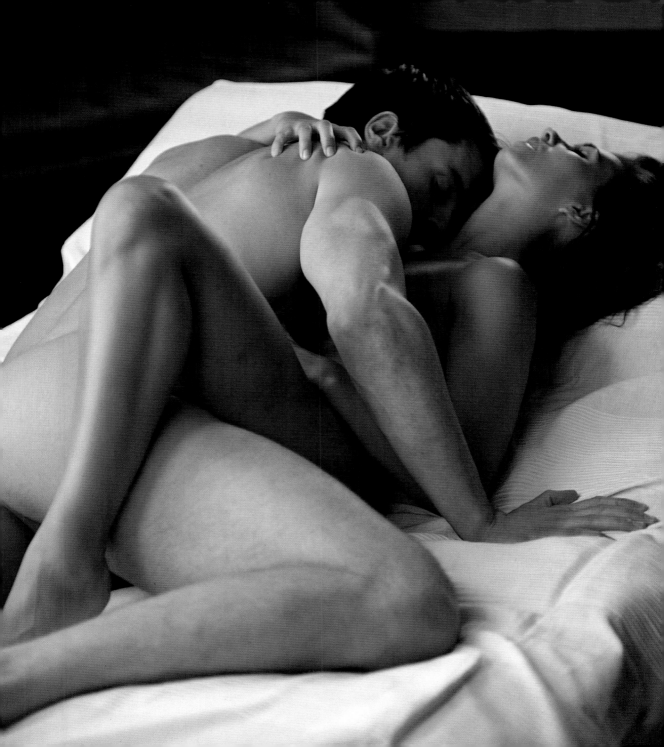

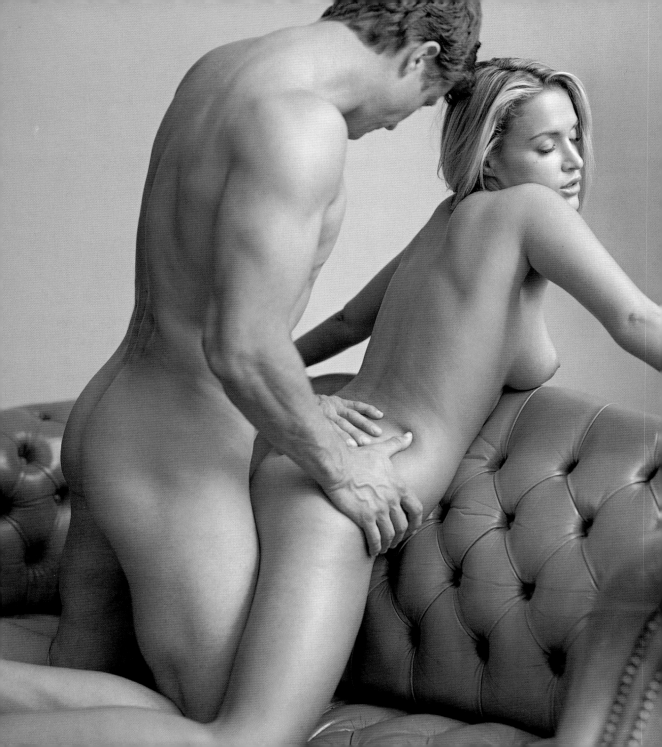

Your orgasms: G-spot

It is thought that stimulating a woman's G-spot can lead to deep, intense orgasms, as well as female ejaculation. As with vaginal orgasms, G-spot climaxes explode along the pelvic and hypogastric nerve system, pulling down the uterus and creating an intense, wide-ranging orgasm.

You on top

Sit on top of your partner, facing his feet while he penetrates you. The angle of your vagina in this position will help his penis to hit the G-spot area directly, and you will be able to control the depth and speed of his thrusting. The G-spot responds best to constant, direct pressure and firm strokes. To vary this, squat on your thighs rather than sit on his lap during penetration. (Strong thighs needed here!)

Doggy style

Kneel on all fours using a bed, chair or stairs for support while your partner stands and penetrates you from behind, holding you by the hips. His penis will be aimed towards the G-spot area more consistently than if you were lying flat on your back. To change the angle and depth of thrusting, move the height of your shoulders or lower yourself onto your elbows.

Need some help?

There is no right way to stimulate the G-spot, and its size and sensitivity varies. You might want to practice on yourself before trying this with your partner, so that you can direct him (see page 32). You also could try a G-spot vibrator, which is specially curved to do the job for you.

Did I just come?

Female ejaculation is a controversial topic. In 1981 researchers Whipple and Perry estimated that around 10 percent of women ejaculate. Later studies have suggested a higher percentage. Pressure on the G-spot can make some women release fluid (usually around a teaspoonful), similar to a man's prostate fluid. It's a totally normal response, but it might take you and your partner by surprise.

Your orgasms: multiple

Ask a woman if she's ever had the pleasure of multiple orgasms, and the answer, unfortunately, will probably be no. It may be that there's a mental block, because we've conditioned ourselves to think we'll only have one orgasm at a time, or that the clitoris is so sensitive after orgasm that it's painful to keep going. But don't give up on the possibility – studies have shown that women are all capable of going from climax to climax!

Lucky for us

Women are more likely to have multiple orgasms than men, who usually need to snooze or at least rest after orgasm. For women, multiple orgasms can come in waves of increasing pleasure, or they can be sequential, when you have one after the other, with some time elapsing in-between. The trick is to stay aroused after the first one.

Manual play

Once you've had an orgasm through solo sex, stop stimulating your clitoris, since it will be very sensitive and probably unable to bear direct stimulation. Stroke your labia and vagina instead for a minute. Then go back to the clitoris and play with it until you feel yourself getting excited again. Keep on fantasizing and thinking about sex. Your second orgasm may feel more intense than the first – or it might be just a flutter.

Oral play

If you've had your first orgasm from intercourse, get your partner to stimulate you orally for a different, more intense sensation – it might be all you need to tip you over the edge again. Take the focus off the clitoris directly and get your partner to work his tongue around the genital area, or inside the vaginal opening, until you're aroused again. He can then go back to direct stimulation of the clitoris. Get him to start out softly and gradually build strokes and pressure as your body responds.

Need help?

Breathe deeply during and after your first orgasm and writhe around to free up your energy. Build up sexual tension by imagining that you are having an orgasm. Try different techniques and work out how long your clitoris needs to recover before you can stimulate it again. Fantasize or watch porn – whatever you need to keep yourself turned on.

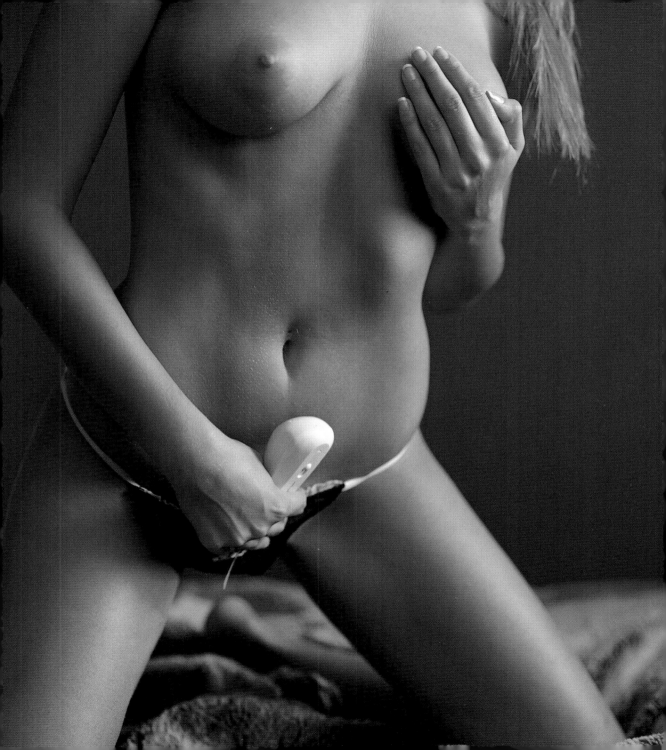

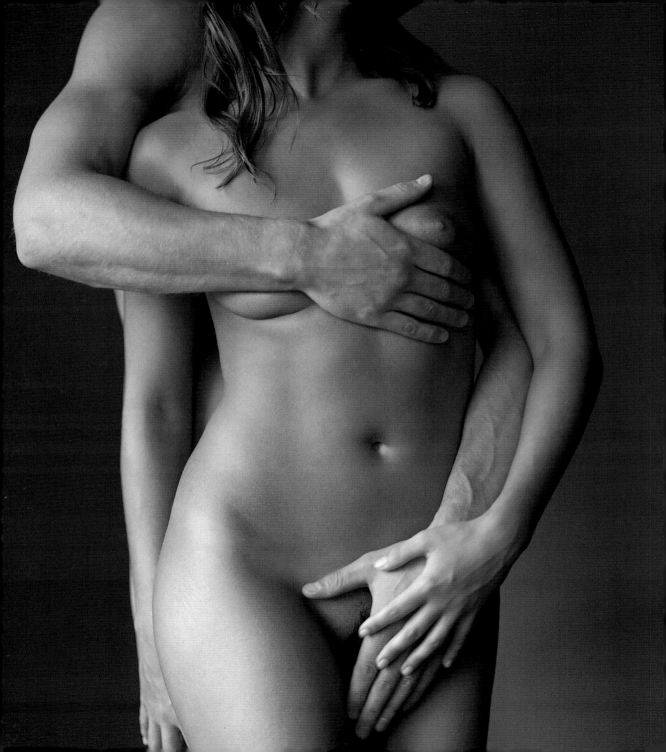

Your orgasms: blended

The term "blended orgasm" was coined by sexologists Whipple and Perry in the 1980s, and basically refers to a sensational mix of the clitoral and vaginal orgasms, which takes place when you stimulate the two areas at the same time. This is one of the most intense orgasms because two different nerve systems are involved: the pudendal for the clitoral climax and the pelvic and hypogastric for the vaginal orgasm.

Manual play

Get your partner to play with your clitoris and G-spot at the same time. Tantric yoni massage is a great way to do this (see page 40). He should use plenty of lubricant and gently circle the clitoris with one hand while using two or three fingers of his other hand to penetrate you. Keep the motion smooth and steady. The experience will be even more intense and erotic if he stimulates your nipples at the same time as your clitoris.

Him on top

If your partner penetrates you vaginally using the coital alignment technique (CAT), both the vagina and clitoris will be stimulated (see page 77). Get him to play with your breasts at the same time, or attach a pair of nipple clamps to stimulate your whole body into a frenzy!

This wonderful combination of clitoral and vaginal orgasms will set your whole body on fire

Doggy style

Ask your partner to stimulate your clitoris or breasts manually while he penetrates you from behind. To really drive yourself crazy, try using a clitoral or nipple sucker at the same time. These are toys that suck at the tip of the breasts or clitoris, replicating the sensation of oral sex. Turn them up and down, varying the speed for a more intense experience.

Your orgasms: anal

Orgasms from anal touching can be very intense for both men and women because of all the different parts of the body that are stimulated. During an anal orgasm, the pelvic muscles surrounding the anus contract, leading to strong sensations all over your vagina and uterus. What's more, double penetration – vaginal and anal – creates an amazingly erotic feeling of fullness. Even if you're not that keen on the idea of anal play, it's worth trying this at least once.

Penetration

The anus is packed with nerve endings and is highly responsive to stimulation. Get your partner to lick around your anal area gently until it relaxes enough for him to penetrate you with a (well-lubricated) finger. If you're worried about hygiene, take a bath first and use a dental dam to cover the area. You can buy these or make your own by cutting a condom in half and placing it between your butt cheeks. This will form a barrier.

Some women love the feeling of being totally "full"

Once the anal sphincter is relaxed and lubricated enough to accommodate his finger, get your partner to keep still inside you while your body gets used to the new sensation. Then he can try inserting the tip of his penis very slowly and gently. The spoons position is a good one for trying anal penetration because it is intimate and relaxing and the anus is accessible. To get you going, your partner can lie behind you for a while, pressing his penis against your vagina and anus.

Need some help?

Try using a butt plug (see page 55) before sex. The anus doesn't lubricate itself, unlike the vagina, so it needs a little assistance. Use a good amount of lubricant and indulge in plenty of foreplay before you insert the plug. Take it easy and you'll be able to achieve a very intense orgasm.

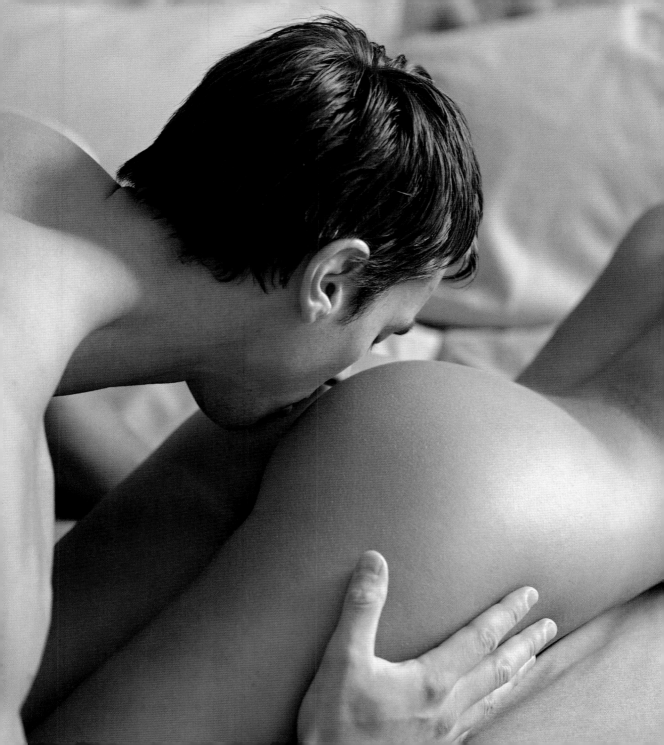

Your orgasms: breasts

Who doesn't love nipple play? It feels very erotic to have your breasts licked, sucked and gently bitten, and the number-one complaint is that men don't do it for long enough! Indulge yourself by devoting a whole evening to the task of reaching an exquisite breast orgasm.

Manual play

Ask your partner to spend at least half an hour playing with your breasts before moving on to anything else. He can vary his technique – stroke, nibble, bite and lick, use ice or candle wax. The idea is to be creative and have fun, focusing on one breast first and then the other. He should keep going until you come. It might be a mini-orgasm, but it's possible! Close your eyes and fantasize while he's doing it to intensify the sensation. If he wants to give you a blended orgasm (see page 85), he can use his other hand to stimulate your G-spot or clitoris at the same time. Alternatively, you can reach down and pleasure yourself.

It is possible to orgasm through nipple play alone – go on, try it!

Need some help?

Wireless vibrating nipple clamps can do the work while your partner is busy elsewhere. He'll probably find it a huge turn-on to see you wearing them. You could ask him to put them on and take them off for you, or to play with your breasts while they're attached. Enhance the sensation by rubbing your nipples while the clamps are attached. Much of the sensation comes when you finally remove the clamps and blood returns to the nipple.

If you find that you're not enjoying the experience, don't worry. Breast play works better at different times of the month. At certain points in your menstrual cycle, your breasts will be sensitive and playing with your nipples may be painful.

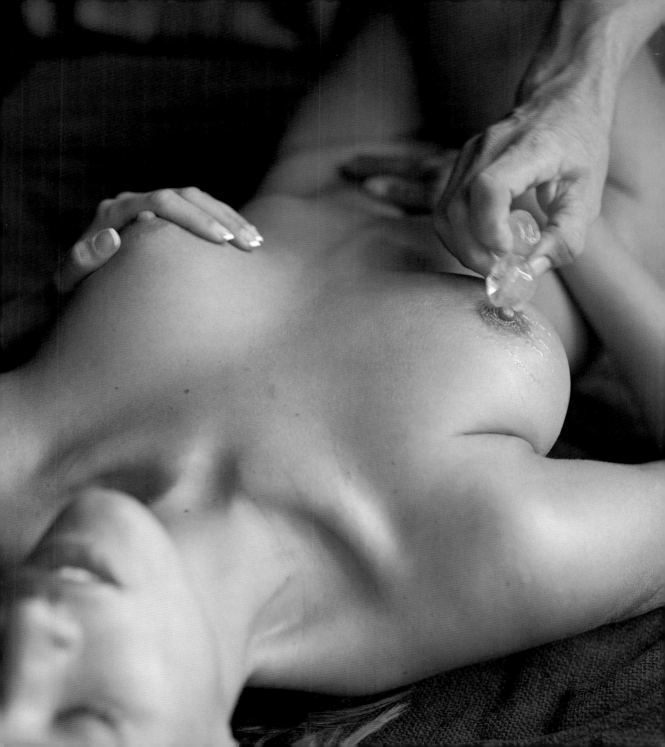

Your orgasms: fantasy

A select few are able to orgasm simply through fantasy – that's right, with no genital stimulation at all! Just think of the possibilities. Kinsey's research in this field was borne out of a 1992 study at Rutgers University showing that fantasy orgasms really do occur.

Mind games

Your imagination is the only limit with this one. Run a bath, relax, touch yourself all over, watch porn or read erotica. Allow yourself to daydream. If there's a sexual scenario that turns you on, embellish it. Letting your imagination run wild is important; the more often you fantasize, the better your orgasms will be. You may find you're more easily turned on at certain times of the month, when extra hormones make your fantasies more intense.

Involve your partner

Ask him to read an erotic story to you or a fantasy you've written yourself. Give him an erotic dance or ask him to perform for you. Create a costume role-play scenario together. When you're feeling turned on, try squeezing your PC muscles tightly. This will awaken the genital area and can trigger orgasm.

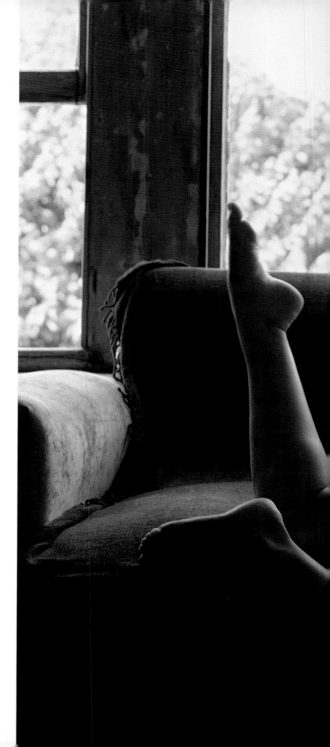

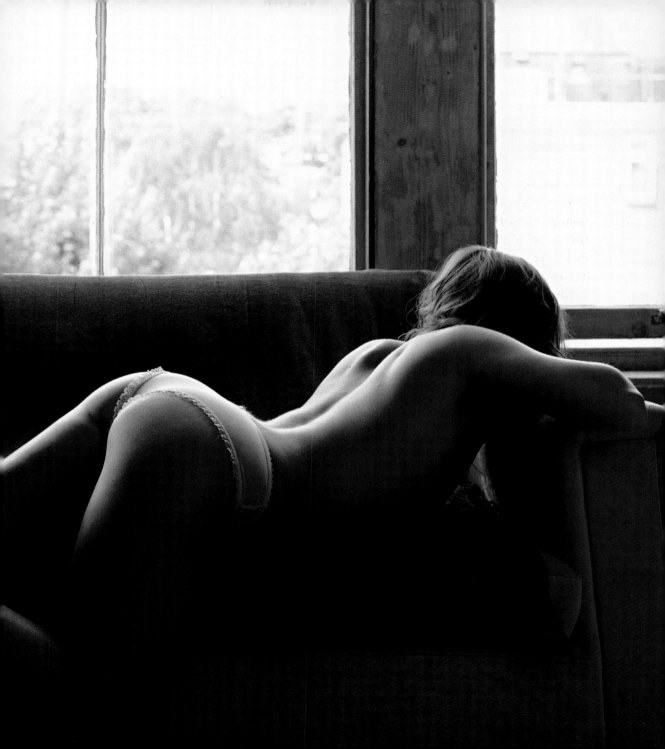

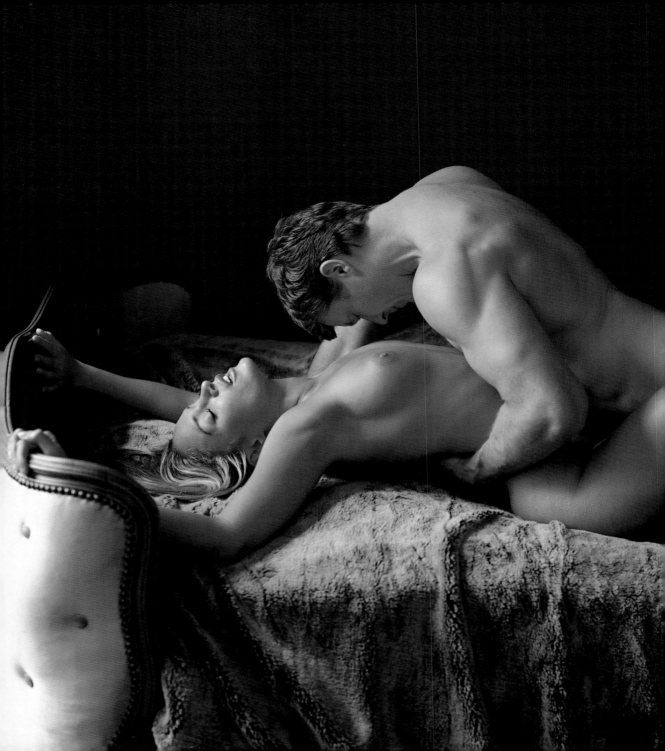

Your orgasms: simultaneous

Having an orgasm at the same time as your partner is a nice idea but, sadly, it rarely happens in real life. This is because it takes you longer to get aroused. By the time you're ready to roll, your partner will probably have come and gone and will have to finish you off! Don't worry if you don't have one. In some ways it's nice to watch him enjoy himself and see what tips him over the edge, then lose yourself in your own ecstasy. There are, however, a few ways in which you can make simultaneous orgasm more probable.

You on top

This position is good for simultaneous orgasm because it puts you in control of the speed and depth of penetration. You can move your body and angle yourself for maximum clitoral stimulation. You can also use a small vibrator on your clitoris, since your hands are free.

Him on top

The CAT variant of the missionary position (see page 77) can work because your partner's pubic bone is connected to yours all the time. He can penetrate you shallowly, rubbing his pubic bone and the base of his penis against your clitoral area in a circular motion. Constant clitoral contact will help you to come more quickly, raising your arousal levels to match his.

Simultaneous orgasms are most likely to happen by chance

Need some help?

If you want to try having an orgasm at the same time, the trick is extended foreplay for you until you're as turned on as he is. Get your partner to give you an erotic massage and then stimulate your clitoris manually or orally. When you come close to orgasm, give him a signal to back off. If he does this several times you will be ready for orgasm as soon as he penetrates you.

Your orgasms: whole body

Sound like bliss? It is! Psychoanalyst Wilhelm Reich first named the whole-body orgasm in the 1920s, theorizing that our bodies and the universe are full of sexual energy. Rather than being focused in the genitals, a whole-body orgasm floods you from head to toe with waves of pleasure. You're probably more likely to have one if you know your body well and keep it sexually charged. Whole-body orgasms are often linked to submissive/dominant play, because an emphasis on experiencing pain and pleasure awakens the entire body.

Wake up the body

Concentrate on stimulating your entire body, not just the genital area. Start with your brain: fantasize, read erotica. Try sensate focus exercises, which are designed to help you and your partner get in touch with your bodies (see page 138). Set aside an evening with your partner to pleasure each other. Touch each other all over – avoiding the genitals at first – to build up sexual energy.

Your entire body becomes one big erogenous zone

Build the tension

When you do move the attention on to your genitals, don't bring each other to orgasm. As soon as you feel yourself getting aroused, he should remove his hands for a minute before playing with you again. When you feel yourself close to orgasm, close your eyes and visualize the climax as a light that fills your entire body. Imagine that you are feeling it in every part of you. By this point, your whole body will be sensitized and your orgasm will be more erotic and powerful than usual. If you practice this approach several times, you will find that over time your climaxes increase in intensity and become totally overwhelming. Tantric sex also explores whole-body orgasm and there are various techniques you can try (see pages 116–121).

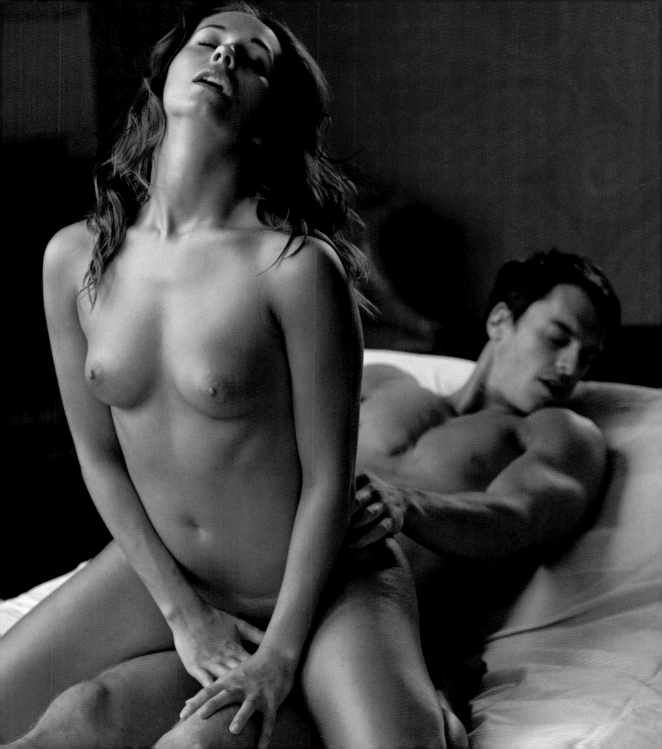

Your orgasms: U-spot

The urethra is surrounded on three sides by your clitoris, so stimulation in this area feels pretty good. You will find your urethra just below the clitoris, above the vaginal opening. It's not the most obvious place to stimulate yourself, since you probably tend to associate it more with peeing than sexual pleasure, but try it and you'll discover a whole new range of delicious sensations!

Oral play

To find your U-spot, your partner needs to open up your inner labia to expose it. He can start by licking it gently, moving around the area. For you to experience a U-spot orgasm, he should continue to apply steady, constant pressure.

You on top

This position works well for U-spot stimulation since it gives you maximum genital contact. During sex, straddle your partner, spreading your legs wide and leaning forwards so that your vulva meets his shaft and pubic bone. This will put pressure on your urethra and gradually bring you to orgasm.

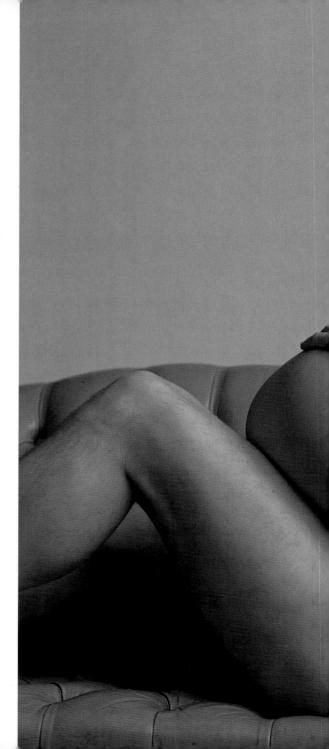

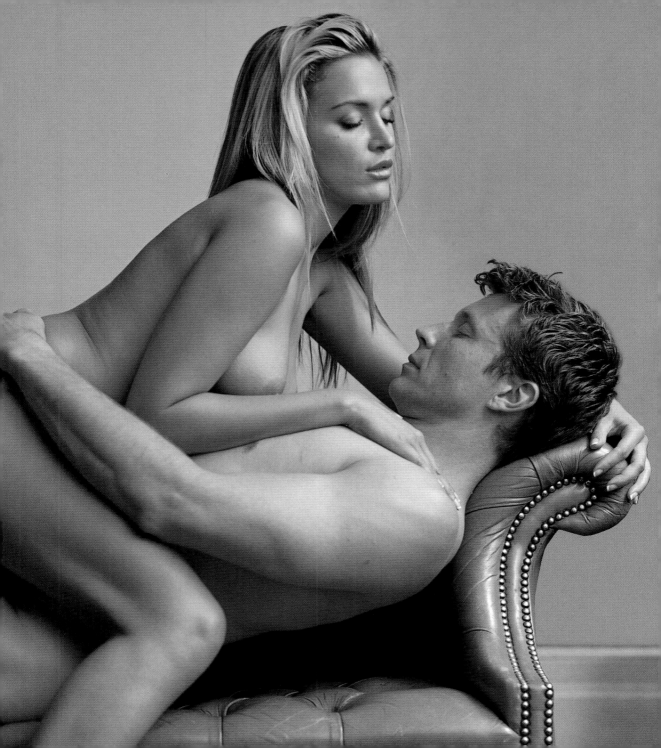

His orgasms: manual

Knowing how to stimulate your partner manually will make you feel sexually confident – and give him no end of pleasure. The best way to learn what does it for him is to watch him while he masturbates. You'll see what he does and how he applies different strokes and varies the pressure to bring himself to orgasm.

A good hand job

Learning how to give a great hand job is a skill worth developing; it will boost your sexual confidence no end. To give your man a truly sensational experience, use plenty of quality lubricant and have your toy box on hand. It's good to experiment with different fabrics to vary the sensation and to keep him guessing. Try out silk scarves, your vibrator, a pearl necklace, your mouth – whatever takes your fancy.

Get his rocks off

Sexologist Lou Paget recommends a technique she calls "Ode to Bryan," so named after a friend who used a spoon to show her what men like! Hold his penis in one hand so that the palm of your hand faces away from you. Your index finger should rest just above his testicles. Move your hand up and down in a steady motion and when you reach the

Blindfold your man so he can't guess your next move

head, imagine that you are twisting open a jar. Keep your hand moving and repeat the motion several times. He will love it when your hand unscrews the jar, so to speak, because the head of the penis is packed with nerve endings and extremely sensitive. Once you partner comes, keep the motion going for a few strokes, rubbing the semen into his penis.

Need some help?

For a different sort of hand job, try the Tantric lingam massage described on page 43, which can be used as foreplay or as a deeply erotic orgasmic experience in itself.

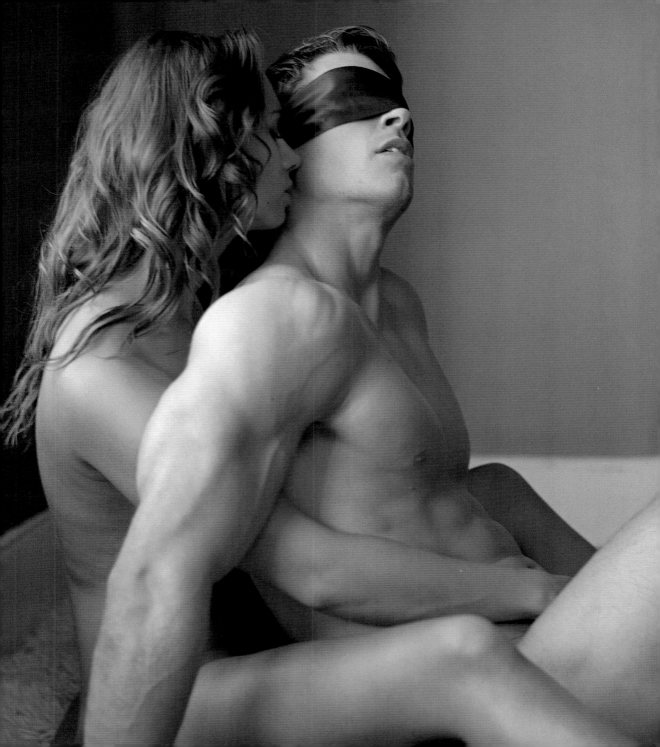

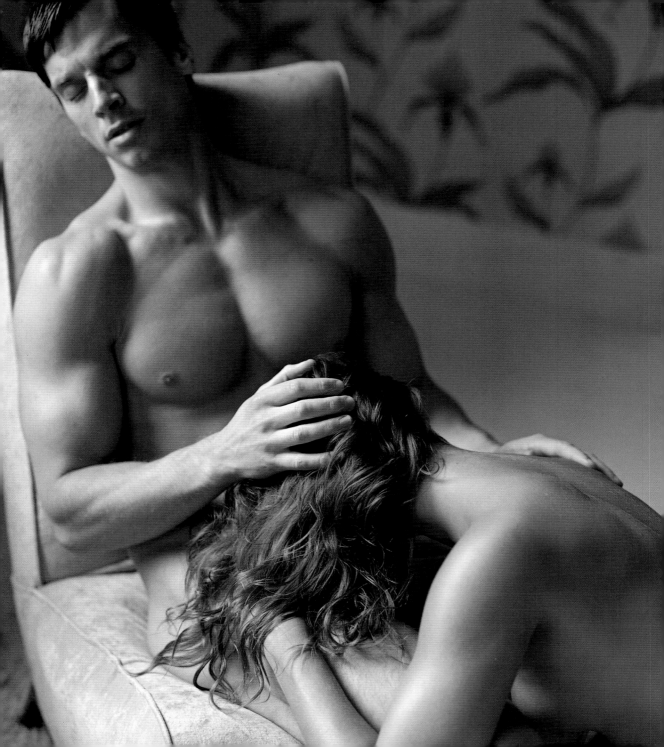

His orgasms: oral

Of all the orgasms, most men rate oral right at the top. Some say that they find oral orgasms even more intense than coming inside their partner. Oral is just so good because your tongue is wet, warm and pliable, and can touch areas that intercourse can't reach. For example, during oral sex it's easier to stimulate his frenulum (the thin strip on the underside of his penis, connecting the shaft to the head) – and the sensation will drive him wild. Read on to discover how to bring your man to oral orgasm (and for more ideas for sexy oral foreplay see page 38).

The killer blow job

Start by running your tongue and hands up and down his shaft a few times to arouse him – don't put his penis into your mouth until he's erect. Then take the head into your mouth. This is the most sensitive part, so if you keep moving away and returning it will feel unbelievably good. Many men like the all-encompassing feeling of being deep-throated. As you pleasure him, remember to keep your jaw slack and teeth behind your lips to avoid biting him. If your mouth gets tired use your hands or a vibrator. Vary the pressure and stroke until you find a rhythm he likes.

When he's about to come, steady, constant pressure works best. He might orgasm more quickly if you also stimulate other body parts. Try playing with his nipples, licking his testicles and scrotum and stimulating his prostate gland. If you don't want him to come in your mouth, get him to give you a signal first so you can finish him off by hand. Most men love it if you swallow – it's kind of dirty and proves that you love every bit of him!

The longer you give head, the more intense his orgasm will be

Need some help?

You are giving your man intense pleasure, and it helps to keep that thought in mind so that you enjoy the experience as much as he does. Visualize his penis as ice cream, licking it in the same way as you would a cone! If you don't like the taste, try using a flavored condom or lubricant. There are also things that you can ask him to do to sweeten the taste of his sperm, like eating strawberries or pineapple beforehand.

His orgasms: anal

The "male G-spot" is his prostate gland, and if he hasn't discovered it yet, he's in for a treat. The prostate is a small gland that's found in his pubic bone, surrounded by pelvic muscles. It responds to pressure through the rectum, externally or internally. When aroused, it releases fluid. If you know how to stimulate this area properly, you'll be able to give him the orgasm of his life.

Manual play

First of all, find out what he likes. Some men prefer having this spot stimulated when they're already turned on, while others find touching it firms up an erection during foreplay. It is located just inside his rectum, so it's easy for you to reach. Use plenty of lubricant, then slowly and gently insert your finger inside his anus (short, clean nails are a must). Once you're inside, stop moving for a moment to give him a chance to get used to the feeling of your finger being in there.

Turbo-charge his climaxes by stimulating the "male G-spot"

Hit the pleasure spot

Now gently move along the wall towards his belly until you find an area that feels a bit like a walnut, 2–3 inches in size. This is his prostate. You'll know when you find it because he'll probably be writhing around in pleasure. Try stroking and touching this area, using different degrees of pressure, until you find out what he likes. Once you've discovered his hot spot, you can stimulate it during sex or while you're giving him a blow job.

Need some help?

If you're a little squeamish about putting your finger up his butt, use a butt plug or an anal vibrator instead (see page 55 for more on boys' toys). Don't worry if your man doesn't like anal play; not all men do and he may find it painful or uncomfortable. If that's the case, leave it and concentrate on pleasuring him elsewhere!

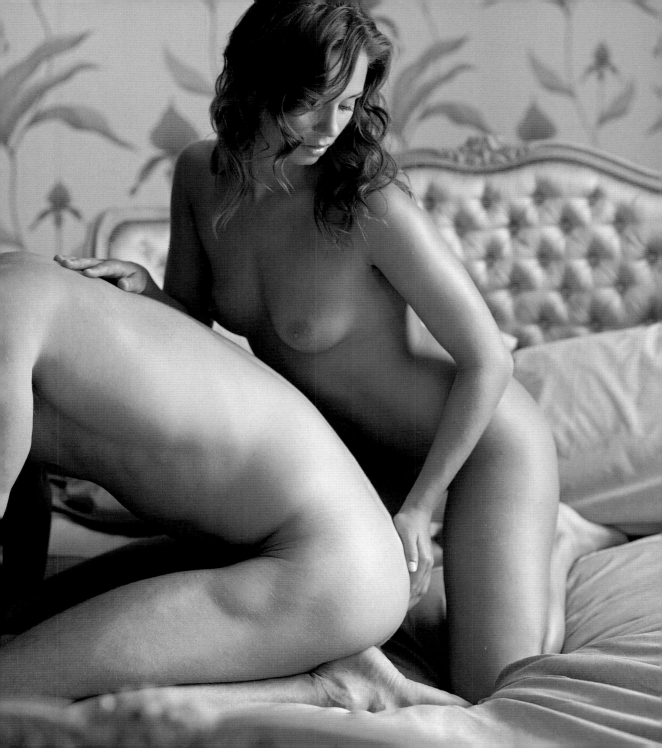

His orgasms: multiple

In 1984, sex researchers Dr. William Hartman and Dr. Marilyn Fithian found that men, like women, are capable of multiple orgasms – although these are rare occurrences. In men, orgasm and ejaculation are two separate responses and the key to multiple orgasms is learning how to control the ejaculate. If he doesn't ejaculate the first time he has an orgasm, he should be able to have another one.

How to do it

Withholding ejaculation is discussed in Eastern sexual traditions, such as Tantra, in which loss of semen is considered to deplete a man's life force. The idea is to circulate ejaculatory energy throughout the whole body rather than dispersing it through the genitals. This can be achieved by strengthening the pubococcygeus (PC) muscles and doing breath work, and there are many books on the subject. Other techniques can help him keep going for longer by temporarily withholding ejaculation (see right). Be aware that persistently holding back ejaculation may put unnatural pressure on the organs, affecting long-term fertility.

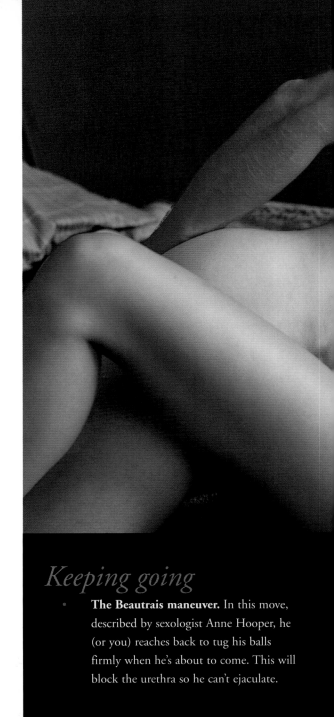

Keeping going

- **The Beautrais maneuver.** In this move, described by sexologist Anne Hooper, he (or you) reaches back to tug his balls firmly when he's about to come. This will block the urethra so he can't ejaculate.

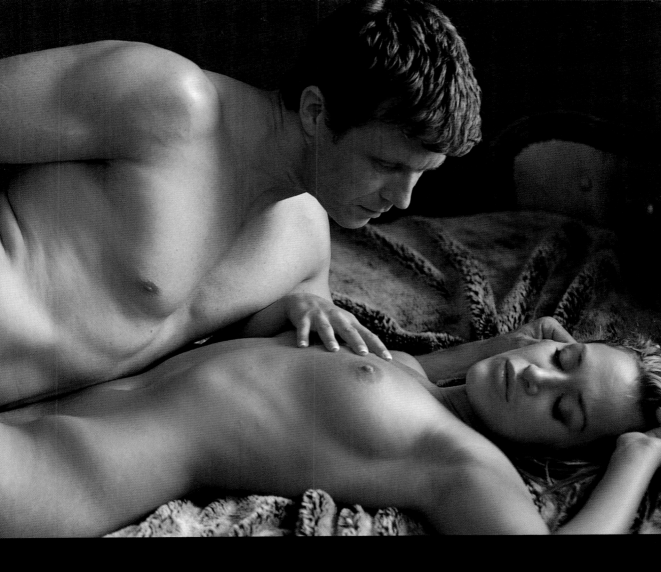

Pressure on the perineum. When he's
about to come, you can put one or two
fingers on his perineum and press inwards
against his pubic bone. This will
effectively block the urethral channel

PC muscle control: If he squeezes his
PC muscles at the point of orgasm he will
orgasm without ejaculating, making it
possible to have another orgasm and/or
more intercourse.

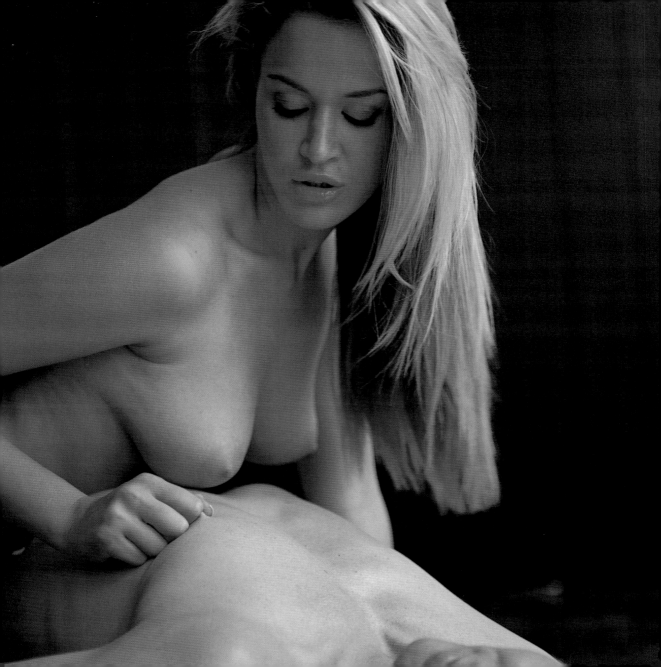

His orgasms: chest

Men don't always care to admit that they love nipple play, perhaps worried that it's a "girl thing." But give it a try: The breast and nipples are full of nerve endings and they respond very quickly to touch, engorging and filling with blood. Like you, your man may experience times of the month where he's more responsive to nipple play than others.

Manual play

Have fun experimenting. Try doing what he does to you when he plays with your breasts and see if it has the same effect. Caress his chest first and then use your tongue to lick his nipples softly. Tug, lick, bite gently or pull them, pull his chest hair and the surrounding area. Use different materials, rough and smooth, hot and cold – such as paper or fabric, wax or ice – for extra sensation. Regular nipple play will give the nipples an enlarged appearance and may enhance their sensitivity.

Lots of men adore nipple play – even if they don't admit it!

Need some help?

If you don't have a pair already, invest in some vibrating nipple clamps, and leave them humming while you attend to other parts. He might not immediately get off on this idea, but for sheer novelty value it has to be worth a try! Be careful not to leave them on for too long, though, since this can cause nerve damage. Remember that he'll feel the most intense sensation when you take them off and blood rushes back to the nipples.

His orgasms: fantasy

As with women, fantasy orgasms are pretty rare for the average man. A survey by Alfred Kinsey in the 1950s showed that out of 5,000 men questioned, fewer than five had experienced an orgasm with no genital stimulation. Still, that doesn't mean it's not worth a try!

Dreamtime fun

Waking fantasy orgasms may be rare, but one very common form of the fantasy orgasm is the wet dream, or nocturnal emission, to call it by its proper name. It is during puberty that boys most commonly ejaculate while they are asleep, but wet dreams can continue into adulthood and men can still experience them in old age. No one really knows why they happen, but theories include sexual desire or a need to release built-up semen. It's thought that they are a common occurrence among men with a high libido – and Kinsey established that women can experience sleep-time orgasms too.

Encourage your partner to stimulate his brain with sexy thoughts and images

Mind games

To help your partner achieve a fantasy orgasm, heat up his imagination by indulging in all sorts of exciting fantasy and sensual thoughts. Turn him on with dirty talk or an erotic story, or do your sexy striptease routine while his hands are tied so he can't touch himself. Men love a visual feast, and he'll probably be turned on by most porn. Tease him as much as you can without giving in. Ask him to describe his favorite fantasy to you – in detail.

Go to town

Go out without any underwear – and let him know when he's least expecting it. Try taking him to a strip club and buying him a few private dances. The sight of naked skin and imagining its touch against his body might just bring your man to orgasm. It could be quite a turn-on for you too.

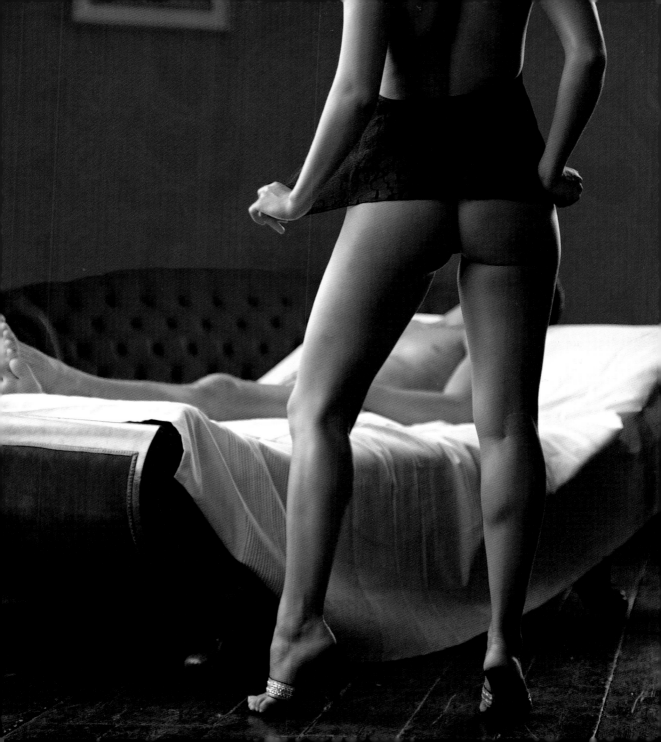

Extended massive orgasm

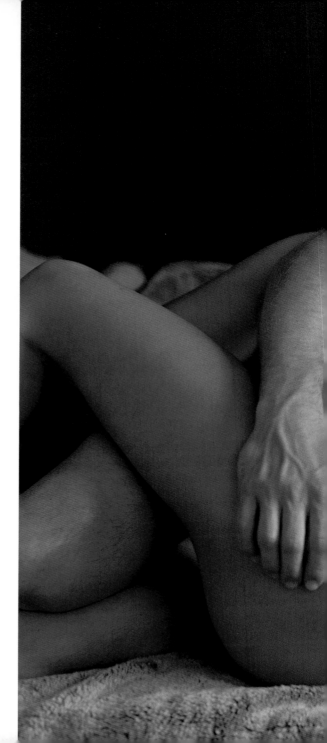

According to sex researchers Steve and Vera Bodansky, it is possible to have an orgasm that lasts anywhere from two minutes to three hours and even longer. Coined the "extended massive orgasm" (EMO), this wonderfully intense orgasm can, it seems, with time and patience, be experienced by anyone, regardless of genetics or luck.

Foreplay is key

In their book *Extended Massive Orgasm* (2000), the Bodanskys describe how to achieve such ecstatic heights. Primarily, it's down to foreplay, mental stimulation and trust. The experience is not actually about the orgasm lasting for three hours, but rather about putting yourself in a state of orgasm and opening your mind to the possibility of it continuing. The more you practice and increase your sexual awareness, the more intense your orgasms will be. Core aspects of the Bodanskys' theories are the exploration of foreplay techniques, getting to know yourself and your body, developing your PC muscles and learning the art of seduction.

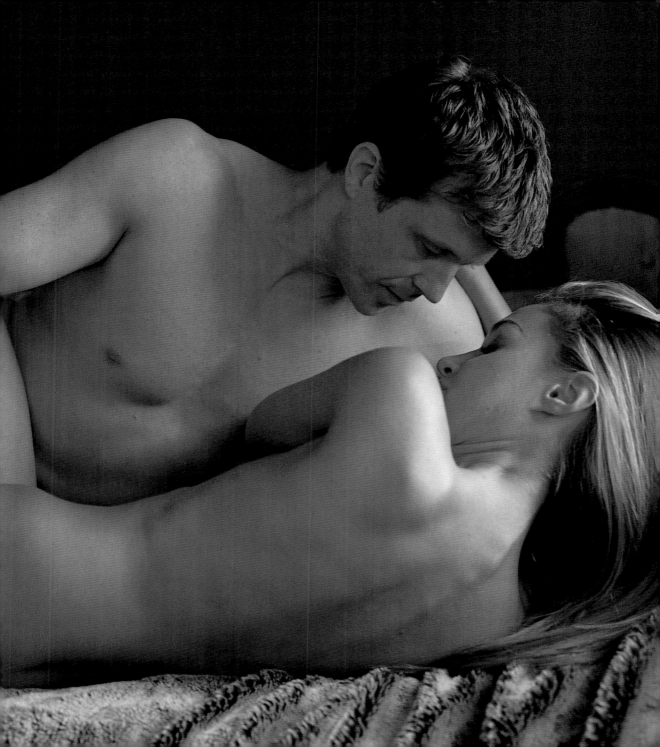

Achieving EMO

There are various approaches to EMO. Start by learning about the different parts of the clitoris and what they do for you. The Bodanskys believe the real magic spot for a woman is the upper left quadrant of the clitoral head – pull back the hood to locate it and trigger amazing orgasms. Massage it gently or get your partner to tease you by gently touching it and backing off until you're worked up to a frenzy. Discover the deep pockets inside the vagina that feel wonderful when they're touched; stimulate your G-spot by yourself or get your partner to do it.

Sensuality exercises

Spend the night tuning into your own pleasure: Take a sensual bath, read an erotic book or magazine and wear sexy fabrics. Make a "visual inventory" (a list of the things you like about yourself) and a "physical inventory" that explores the different ways you like to be touched. Stimulate yourself around your genitals, without touching them directly. Masturbate regularly and practice stimulating two different erogenous areas simultaneously to connect sensations and strengthen your orgasms.

Play

The art of hand-to-genital stimulation is the best way to experience EMO. Lubricate the area well, then explore how and where to touch for the most pleasure, and how to stimulate your G-spot. Try a technique called "dancing on the clitoris," using your fingers to follow a musical beat on your clitoris and rhythmically build up the pleasure.

Peaking

This involves your partner learning how to back off repeatedly, change the rhythm or vary the pressure as you approach orgasm. Reducing and building tension to unbearable levels will finally bring you to an all-consuming orgasm.

Breaks

In the EMO approach, it is important to take regular breaks during sex play. Don't rush towards orgasm, but try stopping and starting to take your partner higher. Communication is also important: Ask each other how you want to be touched.

Relax

Relaxation is key. "Pushing out" is a technique that relaxes the sphincter muscles. Practice it by inserting a small, clean bottle into the vagina when you pee, "pushing out" for a few seconds. You can repeat the motion during sex (without the bottle!).

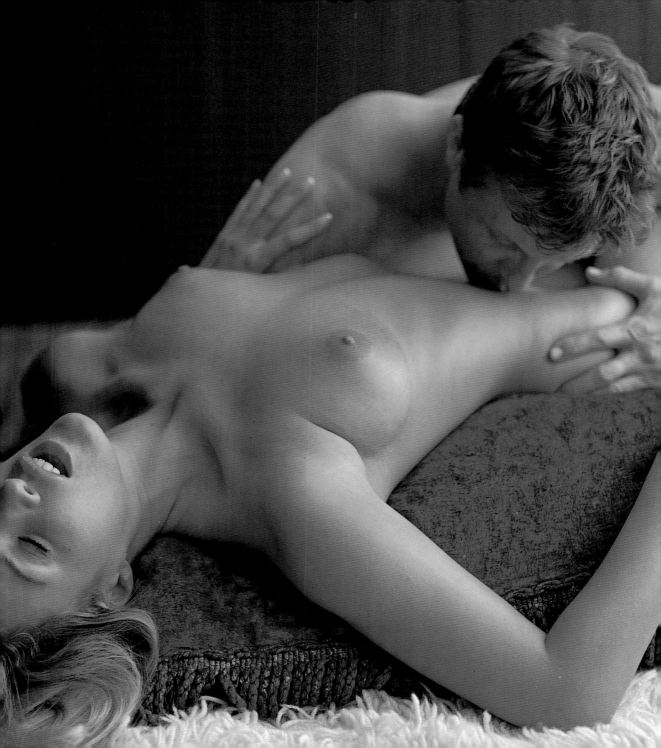

Polynesian slow sex

The Polynesians have an interesting take on sex – a philosophy called slow sex. As recorded by Friedrich Ulvan in the early 20th century, it works on the premise that we are all too focused on orgasm as a goal, and have forgotten the art of sensual touch.

A game of patience

Polynesian slow sex is about taking time to explore each other, so that you arouse your whole body and build up energy or *chi*. In order to preserve sexual energy, you should only have sex once every five days and, in between, should stick to petting and cuddling with no genital contact. When you do eventually have sex you need at least an hour's foreplay and your partner should only penetrate you once your body is fully charged. Once he's inside you, both of you need to relax and resist the urge to move (or laugh) for 30 minutes. You can make small movements if he loses his erection or if you start to lose arousal. Keep your genitals close and connected, and continue to kiss, touch and pleasure each other. When the half hour is over you can move and finally release the pent-up energy. The energy between you both will be amazing, and the orgasm that follows pretty earth-shattering.

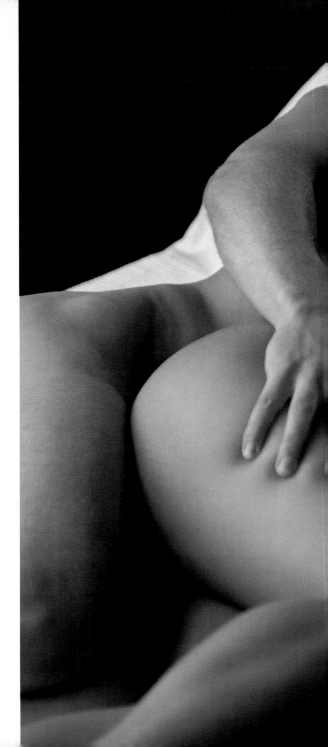

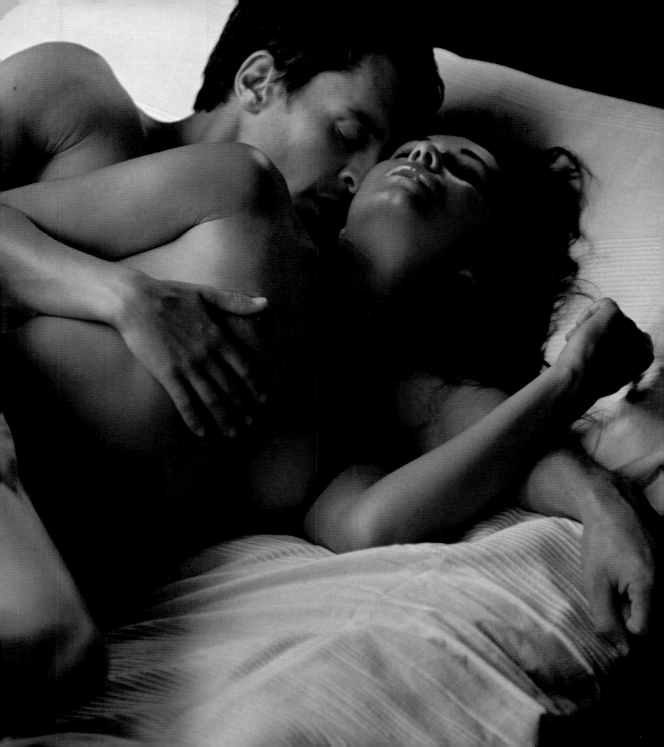

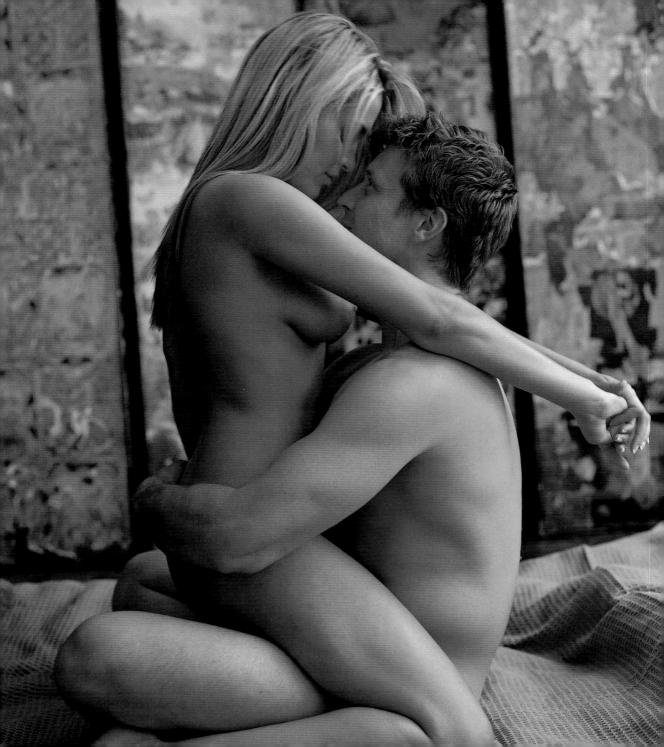

Tantric sex

The word *Tantra* is Sanskrit for "woven together" and it represents an ancient path of self-development that sees sexual energy as the main life force. Followers of Tantra believe that women possess more spiritual energy than men, and that men can join themselves to the divinity through sacred, highly charged, emotional sex with a woman.

Being in the moment

Today, people have many different ideas about Tantra and we tend to associate it most with marathon sex sessions and complicated positions. The basic idea is to stop thinking and to start feeling. Tantra is about being in the moment, with all of your senses aroused; it is an awareness of your sexual energy, being at one with the universe and your partner.

Tantric orgasms are intense and often described as whole-body orgasms. They are not the goal of sex, however; what's important is activating the seven energy centers of the body, the chakras, to reach a higher state of sexual awareness. Being connected to your partner is key. Before you try the Tantric positions, set apart an evening for some exercises to help you connect physically, mentally and spiritually with your partner (see left).

Make the connection

- **Sit opposite** one another with your legs crossed and maintain eye contact.
- **Hold each other's gaze** without letting your eyes wander.
- **Think about the positive feelings** you have for your partner and open your heart to let these flow to him. Enjoy the moment of being connected.

Awaken your senses

- **Blindfold your partner** to sharpen his senses.
- **Play sensual music** or read a fantasy/erotic story to him.
- **Touch him all over** and focus on how he smells.
- **Give a sensual massage** and find out how you like to be touched.
- **Taste each other's bodies** and introduce different foods as part of your sex play.

Tantric positions
for orgasm

Here are some basic Tantric positions. There are many variations, some of which you will doubtless find that you move into naturally. Experiment to add new dimensions to your sex play. You will discover that different postures create a different response in the body.

Yab yum

You sit in his lap with your knees on either side of his body while he penetrates you (see page 116). The classic Tantric pose, this is a cozy and intimate position that leaves you both free to kiss, touch and cuddle as much as you like. It stimulates all seven chakras in both partners, ensuring that you are fully connected to each other. You can touch foreheads and synchronize your breathing to activate the third eye at the top of the head.

Missionary

He lies on top to penetrate you. This position gives your partner great freedom of movement, allowing him to express his sexuality fully and move his lingam freely. It will bring him to orgasm quickly.

In Tantra, orgasms are not the goal of sex, but simply a part of it

Criss-crossed lovers

This is a relaxing yin position, good for helping you to relax into your femininity. Your partner kneels on the bed facing you while you lie flat on your back with one leg across his thigh (see opposite). He can penetrate you gently. This is a good position to try if your partner is not yet fully erect. It is a very intimate, relaxed position, which you can remain in for 20 minutes or so for full benefit.

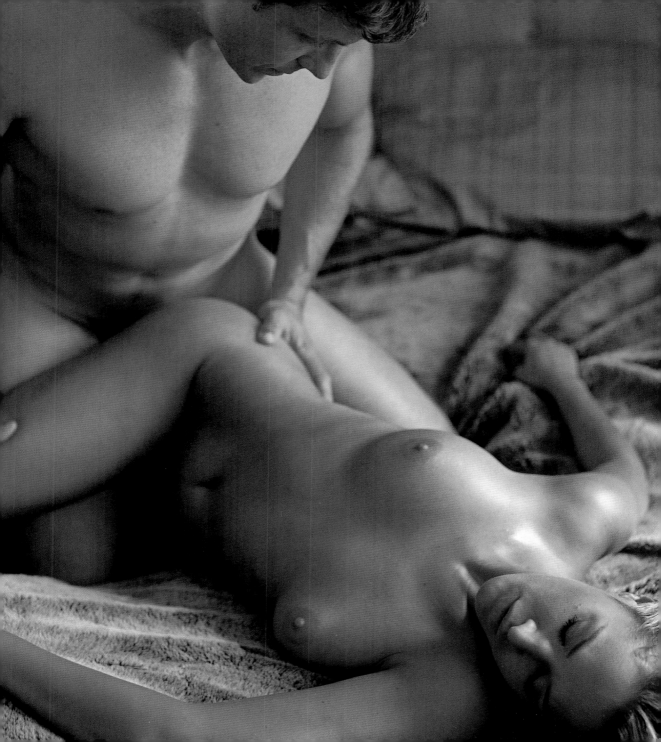

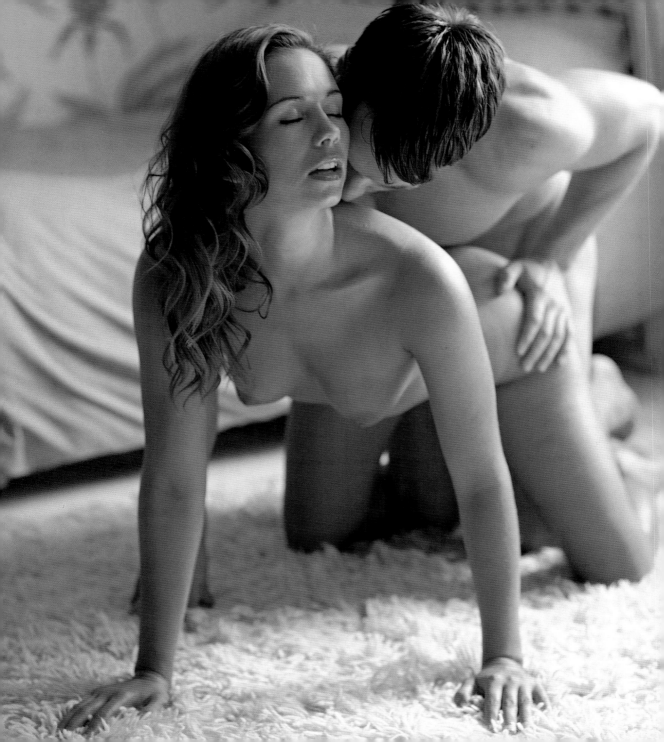

Rear-entry

You crouch on all fours, facing away from him, while he enters you from behind (see opposite). This is a great position for deep penetration. Some women like it because it is very animalistic and allows them to feel totally possessed by their partner. It also gives your partner a fabulous view of your gorgeous butt! Because he can control the depth and speed of penetration, it's important for you to be fully aroused and lubricated to avoid discomfort. Indulge in plenty of foreplay first. You may find this position easier at certain times of the month, according to your hormone levels and the lubrication of your vagina.

Revitalizing

Your partner lies down flat with his legs straight. You sit on his penis, facing his feet, with your chest and head resting along his thighs and toes. This is a good position to try if you're very tired and have been having sex for a while. Stay in the position and recharge your bodies for 15 minutes or so.

A Tantric orgasm fills the body with light and energy

Spooning

You lie on your side with your knees hugging your chest while he mirrors your movements from behind, penetrating you gently. Most of us love spooning since it is an intimate, relaxing and comforting position for both partners. Your partner's hands are free to play with your belly and breasts. A good position for early-morning sleepy sex or just before bedtime.

Praise the goddess

Your partner sits behind you with his legs stretched out straight. You sit on his lap, facing his feet while he penetrates you from behind. This position is very pleasurable for you since it enables your partner to stimulate your clitoris, belly and breasts easily, and to kiss the back of your neck. Being held from behind also feels very protective and nurturing. This position can be calming or vigorous, depending on your mood.

Tao sex

The Tao, a word meaning "the path," is an old Chinese philosophy that harnesses sexual energy to improve health, well-being and relationships. According to Taoist theory, life is a balance of energy forces – yin (female) and yang (male). Men and women need each other's energy to be fully alive and these energies are exchanged during sex. This is known as the "reunion of heaven and earth."

Nine levels

Taoists believe that there are nine levels to a woman's orgasm, and that you need to experience all of them before your sexual spirit can be fully awakened. At the ninth level is the blissful but elusive state of full sexual awakening. Extended foreplay is at the heart of Taoist sexual practice. Only by keeping yourself aroused for as long as possible can you go on to reach the higher levels. Taoist techniques are all about taking your time with foreplay and sex, engaging the senses and all of your body organs – in a way that busy people don't tend to take the trouble to do. It is very easy to let sex slip down the list of priorities; if you don't want to miss out on the most intense experiences, you need to be mindful and make time for pleasure.

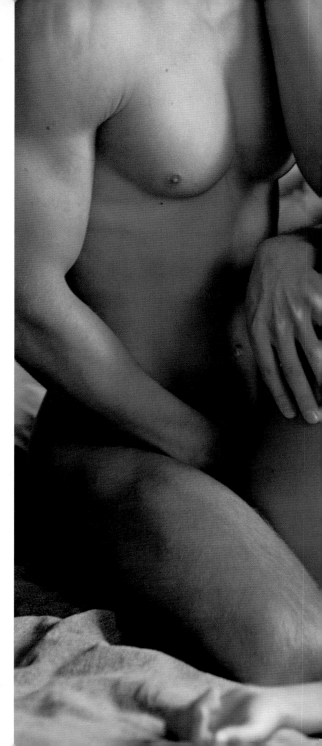

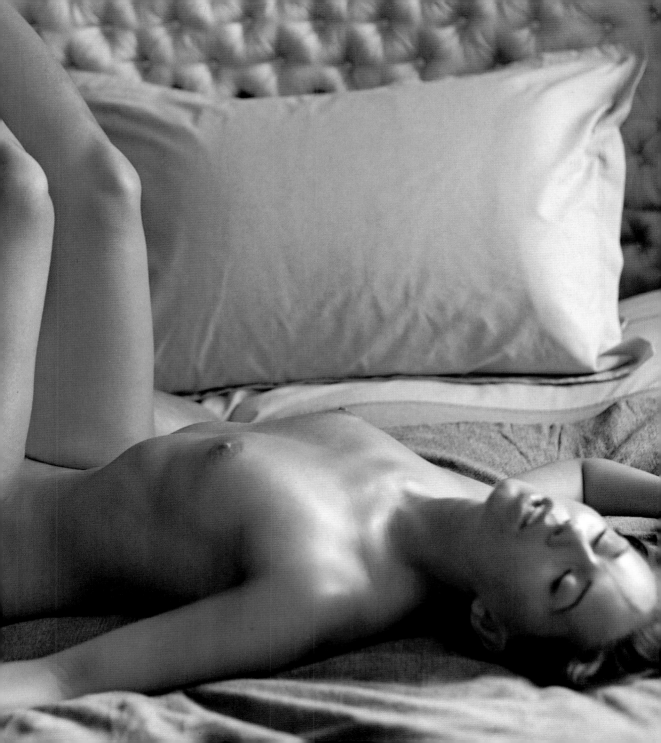

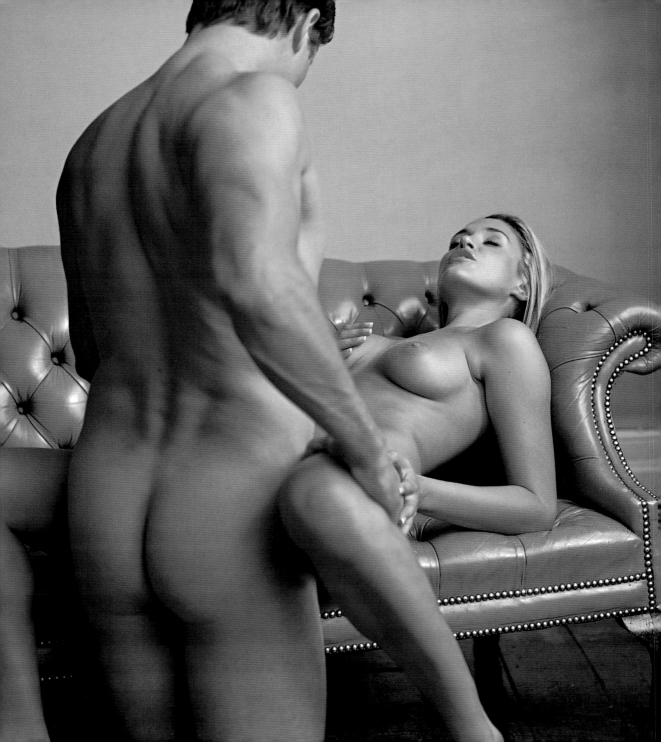

Tao positions
for orgasm

There are many positions in Tao, all of which are simply variations on four basic positions: man on top, woman on top, side to side and rear entry.

The lion hunting

Your partner sits facing you while you lie down on the bed with your legs extended in the air. Supporting your legs with one hand, your partner uses the other to penetrate you (see page 123). This is a good position for deep penetration, so try it once you are fully aroused. You will need additional clitoral stimulation for this position to be enjoyable, since your legs are pretty restricted.

A rose in bloom

This is a variation on the basic missionary position. Your partner is on top while you lie beneath him with your legs wrapped around his back. You can grip his shoulders to change the speed and movement of his thrusting. This position stimulates your clitoris, making it a good position for orgasm.

Eagles in flight

This position is fun because it feels wanton and spontaneous. You lie half on, half off the bed with your legs spread wide, while your partner kneels on the floor and penetrates you (see opposite). Because your bodies are parallel, it will provoke different sensations for both of you. However, there's not much clitoral stimulation so you will enjoy it more if he uses his hands to play with your clitoris.

The birds

Both of you are fully stretched out and you lie on top while he penetrates you. Once he is inside you, both of you extend your arms and hold hands so that you look like birds in mid-flight. This position allows you to dominate, so it is good for letting him relax and experience his yin (feminine) energy.

The snakes

Both of you lie facing each other with your legs stretched out, so that you look like two snakes entwined. He penetrates you and then moves your legs so that they are slightly bent and resting on his thighs (see opposite). This position usually feels better for the woman if the man has a long penis, otherwise it may slip out.

Hunter in the forest

This position allows deep penetration so you will need to be fully aroused before attempting it. You lie on your back and draw your legs towards yourself, so that your ankles are parallel to your chest and your feet are facing the ceiling. Your partner kneels and penetrates you from behind. You are pretty immobile in this position, so make sure you have some clitoral stimulation beforehand.

Taoist sex magic: make a positive wish when you orgasm and it will come true

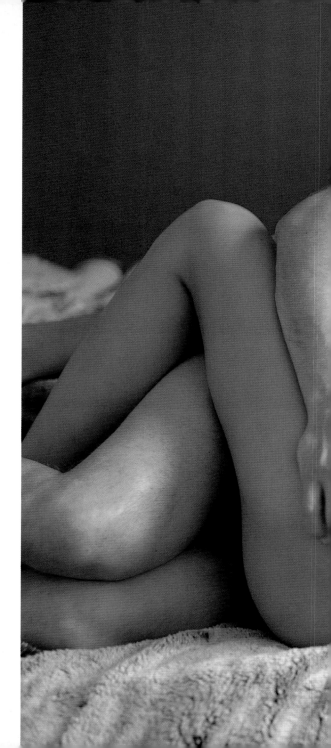

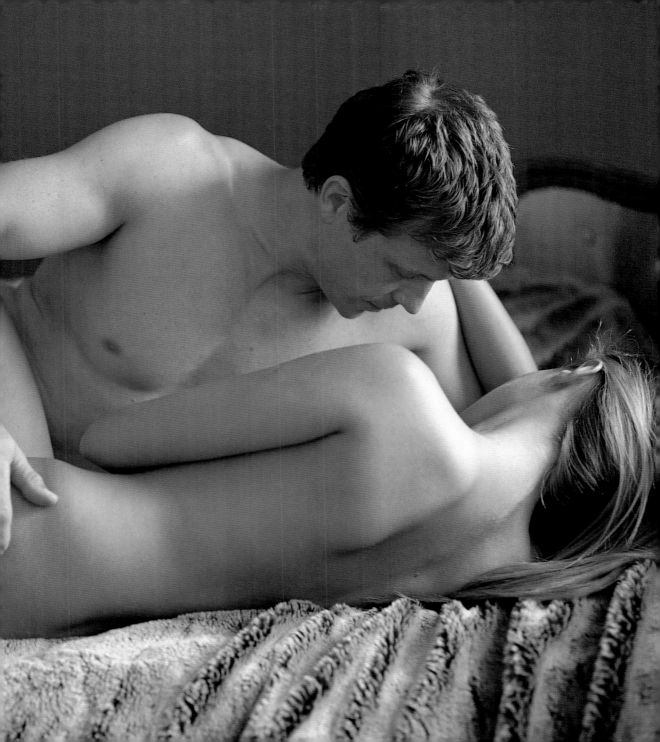

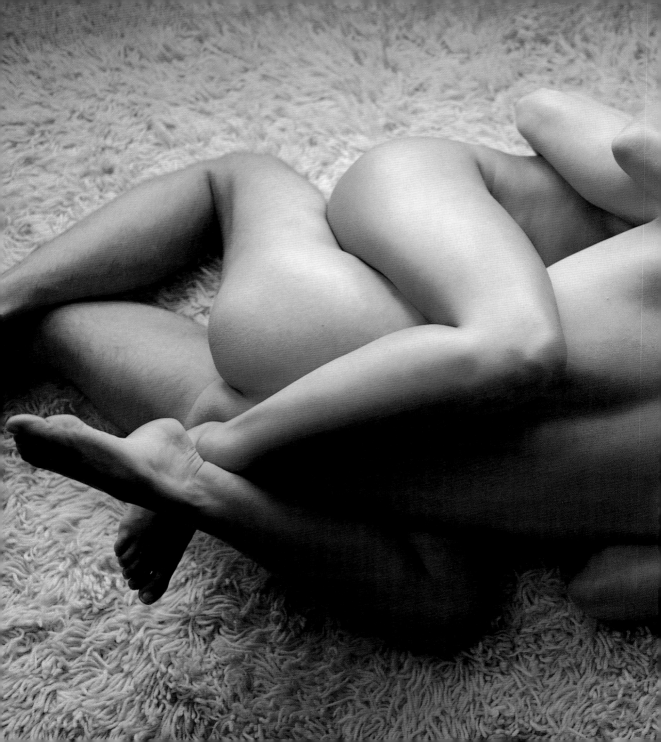

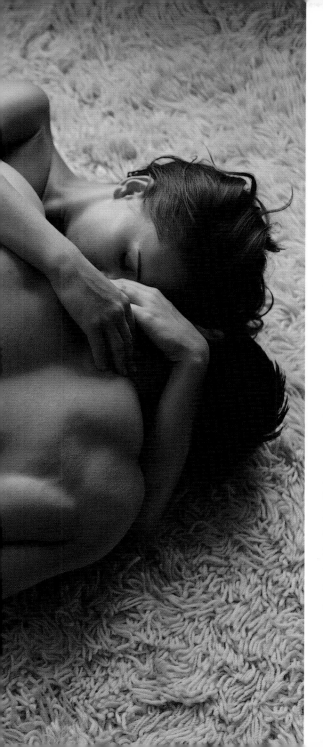

Kama Sutra sex

Written in India some two thousand years ago by the sage Mallanaga Vatsyayana, the *Kama Sutra* was intended as a manual for living for the noblemen of the time. In addition to the detailed explanation of sexual positions that we all know about, the book also explores the art of good manners and human behavior.

Finding balance

The words of the *Kama Sutra*'s title embody the meanings "to enjoy the world" and "spiritual teaching," and so refer to achieving a balance of the physical and spiritual in life. Although it was aimed at men, there are many tips for enhancing female pleasure, so it's definitely worth exploring the book's seven sections, each one written by an expert in the field. The topics covered range from foreplay, orgasms and sex positions to discussions on the nature of love, the art of seduction and the use of herbs, aphrodisiacs and love spells.

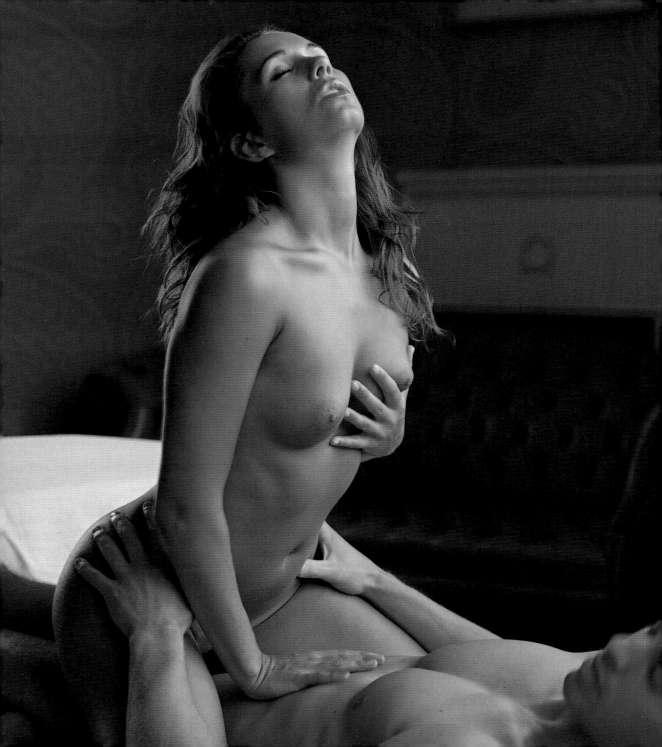

Kama Sutra positions for orgasm

In case you were wondering, the Kama Sutra lists 64 sexual positions. Vatsyayana thought that there were eight ways of making love, each one multiplied by eight possible positions. In the book he calls these positions the "64 arts."

The vines

Both of you lie on your sides facing each other with your arms and legs entwined (see pages 128–29). Your partner penetrates you. He can bend his legs to make this deeper. This is an intimate, cozy position that allows full-body and face-to-face contact.

The Kama Sutra is probably the most famous book about sensual pleasure ever written

Surfing the wave

Your partner lies on his back and you kneel over him with your legs wrapped around his (see opposite). You control the speed and depth of penetration in this position, moving from side to side as well as up and down to stimulate yourself fully. This should bring him to orgasm pretty quickly since he can lose himself while you are doing most of the hard work!

Tiger crouching

You sit on your partner's penis, facing away from him, while he sits with his legs stretched out. You have the flexibility to move and he can support you by lifting your butt and thighs. To vary this position, your partner can use a wall for support and you can kneel rather than sit to alter the angle of penetration. This is a good rear-entry position for you, since it allows you more movement than usual. Your partner can also play with your breasts and clitoris. This one can be very tiring for him!

The arc

Your partner lies flat on his back and you sit on top
of his penis, facing his feet (see opposite). Once he
is inside you, you can lean backwards, supporting
yourself with both arms, so that your hair tickles his
chest. You move up and down. This position is
adventurous and agile, giving you full control of the
speed and depth of penetration. It is very tricky to
maintain, however, since it is easy for him to pop out.

Spider's web

This is a fun, sexy position that can be taken out of
the bedroom. You sit on the end of the bed or on a
chair while he kneels in front to penetrate you.
Once he is inside you, you wrap your legs around
his for balance and deeper penetration. You can also
vary the height of this position by sitting on a table
while he stands in front.

Wings of a plane

You lie on top of him with your legs open so that
he can penetrate you. When he is inside, both of
you straighten your bodies so that you are lying
parallel, in harmony. Provide extra stimulation by
moving your body up and down. This position gives
good body contact and it will feel intense for both
of you because your vagina grips him tightly.

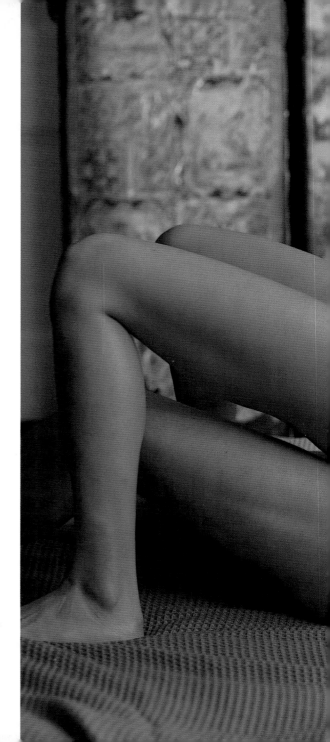

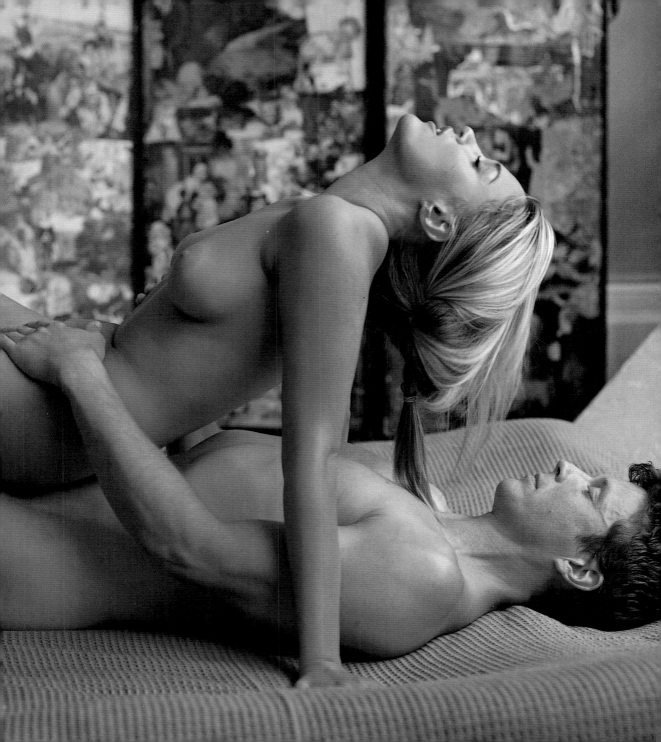

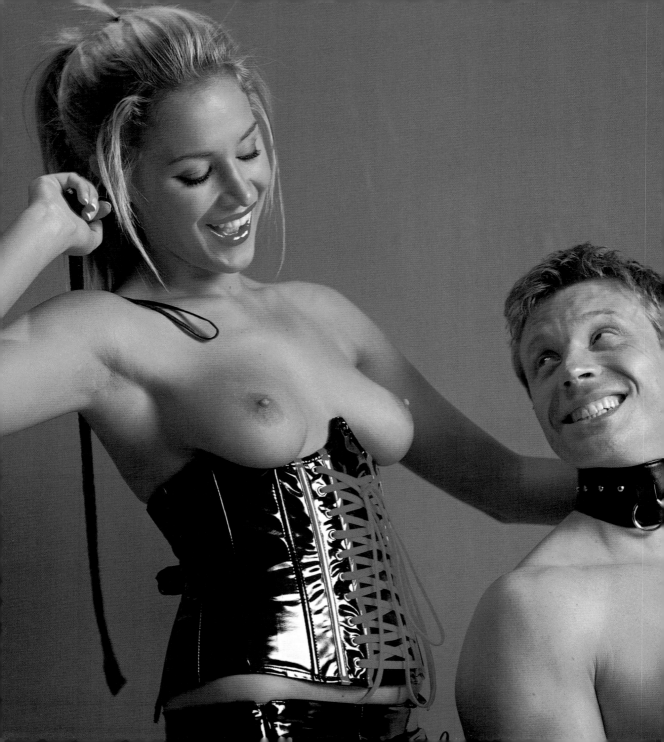

Get out of **that rut**

It is very easy to fall into a sex rut once the passion of a new relationship wears off and you settle down into cozy coupledom. Work, children, lifestyle and stress can all impinge on your sex drive. If you're having sex once a month and that's okay for both of you then it's not an issue. It only becomes one if it starts to bother you or affect your relationship.

Spice it up

Most couples settle into a sex routine where they have one or two favorite positions and tend to have sex at the same time of day when it's convenient. Studies have also shown that couples have less sex the longer they are together. That doesn't mean it has to be poor sex: In fact, longer-term couples tend to have more inventive, satisfying sex, probably because they know each other's bodies so well. If you feel your sex life could do with a little extra spice, there are a few things you can try.

Move over, darling

Try new positions. Most couples settle into the favored one or two because they are tried and tested and bring you (or him) to orgasm quickly. There are lots of books out there that explore sexual positions and you can have fun trying out a few new techniques – even if you never do them again. If you always have sex in bed, move to a different location and vary the times of day.

Make time for sex

Keep your relationship fresh by going away once a month, eating out regularly and getting someone to take the kids (if you have any) so that you can enjoy a night of sensual bliss together. Make sure you communicate properly, keep flirting, touching and kissing. Learn how to give a good erotic massage. Have more sex and initiate it even if you don't feel like it – the more orgasms we have, the more our bodies want.

Fantasy

Go to town with your toy box – there are plenty of innovative sex toys out there to pleasure different parts of your body (see pages 52–55). Try new lubricants – they really make things move more smoothly. Experiment with sexy underwear, fantasy costumes and role play. There are plenty of alternative lifestyles out there if you're curious to stretch your boundaries – swinging resorts, hotels, fetish clubs and naturism, to name a few.

Spend time apart

There's something to be said for not seeing your partner for a few days: It will make you both appreciate each other and sex that little bit more. Try to have a few special interests that you pursue on your own; if you do exciting things separately you'll have more to talk about and your time together will be that much more special.

Exercise regularly

Exercise puts you in a good mood, raises the endorphins and makes you more likely to want sex. It also has the added benefit of making you feel more sensual and body confident. A good half-hour's workout three times a week is all you need.

Eat well

Your body needs a nutritious balance of vitamins, minerals and the different food groups in order to function sexually. Experiment with aphrodisiacs, herbal supplements and cut down your fat, meat and alcohol intake. A diet that's high in fat and cholesterol makes you feel sleepy and sluggish so the last thing you'll feel like doing at night is having sex. Experiment with food play during sex too.

Body modification

There's something out there for everyone. Most piercings are done to enhance sexual pleasure. A ring that runs through the top of a man's urethra on the penis head and emerges underneath the shaft is said to increase stimulation to the clitoris during sex. Female genital piercings are usually at the base of the vagina or behind the clitoral hood. Nipple piercing is another option to increase your sensitivity.

Pubic experiments

Shave off all of your pubic hair for a different sensation during oral sex and intercourse. Or, go for one of the latest crazes – Brazilian, Hollywood or the Tiffany Box (in which everything is shaved off apart from a tiny square, which is then dyed blue to match the color of jeweler's gift boxes). It's good for a giggle if nothing else.

Be prepared

Make sure you always have condoms, lubricant and sex toys on hand – wherever you are. Keep them in your handbag, in the car, in different places around the house. Sex will become spontaneous and adventurous, and you'll find yourself getting into the mood at the oddest times of day…

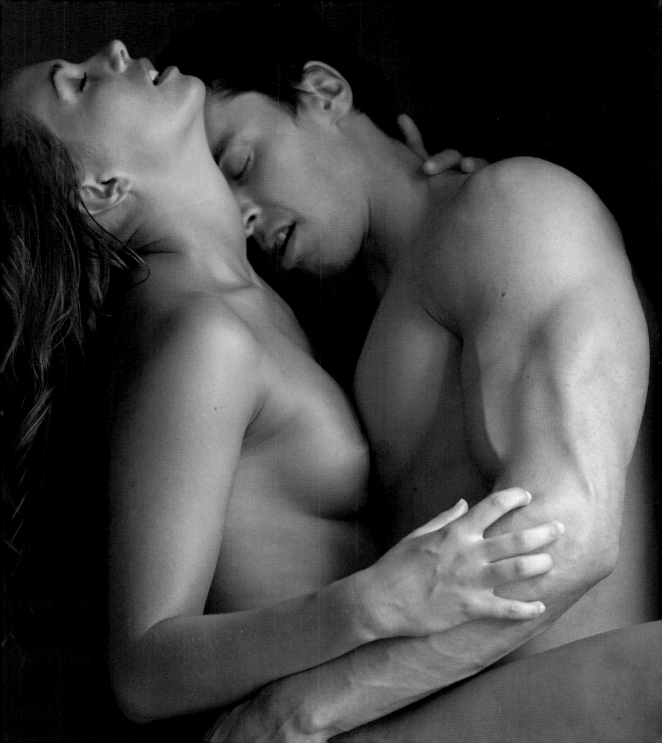

Solving problems

The difficulties outlined at the beginning of this book (see pages 20–23) can be the cause of much tension and stress in a relationship, and should not be left untreated. You may think you and your problem are unique, but you are wrong and, in most cases, there is a solution within reach.

Physical solutions

The first step is to see your doctor to rule out anything physical. Anorgasmia sufferers may discover that they have poor blood circulation, weak PC muscles or a spinal injury that interferes with their ability to orgasm. For sufferers of vaginismus, women might resolve the problem by applying simple relaxation techniques or using vaginal trainers to recondition the PC muscles. It will also help to discuss both problems with a sex therapist (see below).

Physical causes of erectile dysfunction include deficient blood flow to the penis, hormone problems or diabetes, all of which can be treated. Diet and drinking or smoking habits may also contribute, in which case it makes sense to adopt a few lifestyle changes. Sufferers of premature ejaculation can try a start-stop technique of stimulating the penis then easing off, and repeating, in order to recognize the point of ejaculation and practice how to delay it.

Psychological solutions

If the issue is psychological in nature you can seek further help from a counselor or sex therapist. Sex therapy is a very effective way of treating most sexual dysfunctions and is something that you can do alone or with your partner at your own pace. Your therapist will ask you about your sexual history, relationships, attitudes and feelings towards sex, and your specific problem. He or she will then discuss possible causes and suggest treatment methods. You may be given exercises to do, such as sensate focus exercises, which you can do alone and with your partner. These involve touching each other in a non-sexual way to begin with, then gradually building up to sex when you are ready. This form of foreplay can help you get to know your bodies and take pleasure from them. Best of all, it takes the focus off penetrative sex and orgasm and therefore reduces much of the tension that causes the problem in the first place.

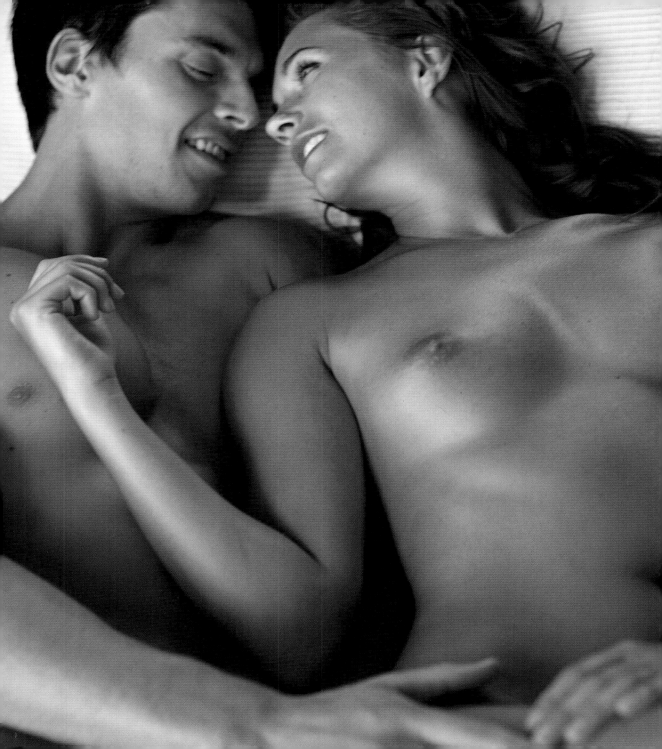

Female and male anatomy

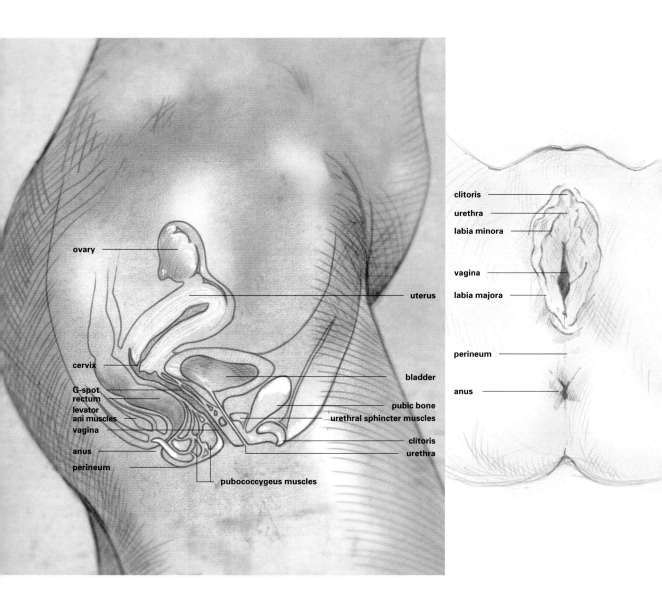

ovary

uterus

clitoris
urethra
labia minora

vagina

labia majora

cervix

bladder

G-spot
rectum
levator
ani muscles
vagina

pubic bone
urethral sphincter muscles

perineum

clitoris
urethra

anus

anus
perineum

pubococcygeus muscles

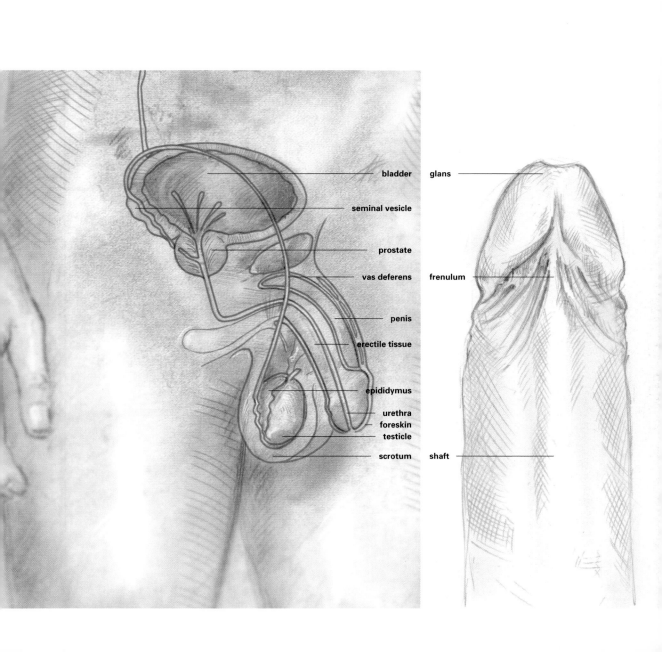

bladder

seminal vesicle

prostate

vas deferens

penis

erectile tissue

epididymus

urethra
foreskin
testicle

scrotum

glans

frenulum

shaft

Index

Acknowledgments

Executive Editor Jane McIntosh
Project Editor Fiona Robertson
U.S. Proofreaders Elyce Petker, Lily Chou

Executive Art Editor and Design Darren Southern
Photography John Davis/© Octopus Publishing Group Ltd
Cover Design DiAnna VanEycke

Senior Production Controller Martin Croshaw